THIS BOOK BELONGS TO:

CONTACT INFORMATION	
NAME	
ADDRESS	
PHONE #	
EMAIL	

Copyright © Teresa Rother
All rights reserved. No part of this publication may be reproduced, distributed, or transmitted in any form or by any means, including photocopy, recording, or other electronic or mechanical methods.

DEDICATION

This Hot Sauce Tasting Journal is dedicated to people who love spicy, fiery food and want to document their findings.

You are my inspiration for producing this book and I'm honored to be a part of your record-keeping and organization.

HOW TO USE THIS BOOK

This Hot Sauce Tasting Journal will help you by accurately recording and organizing your information.

Here are examples of information for you to fill in and write the details of your logbook.

Fill in the following information:

1. Name, Brand, Origin - Record hot sauce information.
2. Sampled - Record where you sampled the product.
3. Scoville - Use the Scoville heat scale and record the number.
4. Texture and Color - Write down how you viewed the texture and color.
5. Heat - Use the chart to describe the heat from mild to extreme
6. Flavor - Use the chart to describe the flavor (fruit, floral, salty, sweet, etc.).
7. Heat Level - Rate the heat level 1-10.
8. Main Ingredients - Write down some of the main ingredients.
9. Additional Notes - Use this space to write additional information.
10. Would You Buy It Again? - Answer yes or no to the question.
11. Overall Rating - Use the rating scale __/10 to record the overall rating.

HOT SAUCE TASTING JOURNAL

NAME		BRAND	
ORIGIN		SAMPLED	
SCOVILLE		TEXTURE	
COLOR		PRICE	

HEAT

○ MEH	○ MILD
○ MEDIUM	○ HOT
○ VERY HOT	○ POWERFUL
○ PAINFUL	○ EXTREME

FLAVOR

○ LINGER	○ BERRY FRUIT	○ CITRUS FRUIT	○ TROPICAL FRUIT
○ DARK FRUIT	○ FLORAL	○ HERBAL	○ VEGETAL
○ GARLIC/ONION	○ VINEGAR	○ SALTY	○ SWEET
○ SPICES	○ SMOKY	○ ROASTY	○ CHOCOLATE

HEAT LEVEL

○ 1	○ 2	○ 3	○ 4	○ 5	○ 6	○ 7	○ 8	○ 9	○ 10

MAIN INGREDIENTS

ADDITIONAL NOTES

WOULD YOU BUY IT AGAIN?		OVERALL RATING
○ YES	○ NO	/ 10

HOT SAUCE TASTING JOURNAL

NAME		BRAND	
ORIGIN		SAMPLED	
SCOVILLE		TEXTURE	
COLOR		PRICE	

HEAT	
○ MEH	○ MILD
○ MEDIUM	○ HOT
○ VERY HOT	○ POWERFUL
○ PAINFUL	○ EXTREME

FLAVOR			
○ LINGER	○ BERRY FRUIT	○ CITRUS FRUIT	○ TROPICAL FRUIT
○ DARK FRUIT	○ FLORAL	○ HERBAL	○ VEGETAL
○ GARLIC/ONION	○ VINEGAR	○ SALTY	○ SWEET
○ SPICES	○ SMOKY	○ ROASTY	○ CHOCOLATE

HEAT LEVEL									
○ 1	○ 2	○ 3	○ 4	○ 5	○ 6	○ 7	○ 8	○ 9	○ 10

MAIN INGREDIENTS

ADDITIONAL NOTES

WOULD YOU BUY IT AGAIN?		OVERALL RATING
○ YES	○ NO	/ 10

HOT SAUCE TASTING JOURNAL

NAME		BRAND	
ORIGIN		SAMPLED	
SCOVILLE		TEXTURE	
COLOR		PRICE	

HEAT

○ MEH	○ MILD
○ MEDIUM	○ HOT
○ VERY HOT	○ POWERFUL
○ PAINFUL	○ EXTREME

FLAVOR

○ LINGER	○ BERRY FRUIT	○ CITRUS FRUIT	○ TROPICAL FRUIT
○ DARK FRUIT	○ FLORAL	○ HERBAL	○ VEGETAL
○ GARLIC/ONION	○ VINEGAR	○ SALTY	○ SWEET
○ SPICES	○ SMOKY	○ ROASTY	○ CHOCOLATE

HEAT LEVEL

○ 1   ○ 2   ○ 3   ○ 4   ○ 5   ○ 6   ○ 7   ○ 8   ○ 9   ○ 10

MAIN INGREDIENTS

ADDITIONAL NOTES

WOULD YOU BUY IT AGAIN?		OVERALL RATING
○ YES	○ NO	/ 10

HOT SAUCE TASTING JOURNAL

NAME		BRAND	
ORIGIN		SAMPLED	
SCOVILLE		TEXTURE	
COLOR		PRICE	

HEAT			FLAVOR			
○ MEH	○ MILD		○ LINGER	○ BERRY FRUIT	○ CITRUS FRUIT	○ TROPICAL FRUIT
○ MEDIUM	○ HOT		○ DARK FRUIT	○ FLORAL	○ HERBAL	○ VEGETAL
○ VERY HOT	○ POWERFUL		○ GARLIC/ONION	○ VINEGAR	○ SALTY	○ SWEET
○ PAINFUL	○ EXTREME		○ SPICES	○ SMOKY	○ ROASTY	○ CHOCOLATE

HEAT LEVEL

○ 1   ○ 2   ○ 3   ○ 4   ○ 5   ○ 6   ○ 7   ○ 8   ○ 9   ○ 10

MAIN INGREDIENTS

ADDITIONAL NOTES

WOULD YOU BUY IT AGAIN?		OVERALL RATING
○ YES	○ NO	/ 10

HOT SAUCE TASTING JOURNAL

NAME		BRAND	
ORIGIN		SAMPLED	
SCOVILLE		TEXTURE	
COLOR		PRICE	

HEAT

○ MEH	○ MILD
○ MEDIUM	○ HOT
○ VERY HOT	○ POWERFUL
○ PAINFUL	○ EXTREME

FLAVOR

○ LINGER	○ BERRY FRUIT	○ CITRUS FRUIT	○ TROPICAL FRUIT
○ DARK FRUIT	○ FLORAL	○ HERBAL	○ VEGETAL
○ GARLIC/ONION	○ VINEGAR	○ SALTY	○ SWEET
○ SPICES	○ SMOKY	○ ROASTY	○ CHOCOLATE

HEAT LEVEL

○ 1   ○ 2   ○ 3   ○ 4   ○ 5   ○ 6   ○ 7   ○ 8   ○ 9   ○ 10

MAIN INGREDIENTS

ADDITIONAL NOTES

WOULD YOU BUY IT AGAIN?		OVERALL RATING
○ YES	○ NO	/ 10

HOT SAUCE TASTING JOURNAL

NAME		BRAND	
ORIGIN		SAMPLED	
SCOVILLE		TEXTURE	
COLOR		PRICE	

HEAT			FLAVOR			
○ MEH	○ MILD		○ LINGER	○ BERRY FRUIT	○ CITRUS FRUIT	○ TROPICAL FRUIT
○ MEDIUM	○ HOT		○ DARK FRUIT	○ FLORAL	○ HERBAL	○ VEGETAL
○ VERY HOT	○ POWERFUL		○ GARLIC/ONION	○ VINEGAR	○ SALTY	○ SWEET
○ PAINFUL	○ EXTREME		○ SPICES	○ SMOKY	○ ROASTY	○ CHOCOLATE

HEAT LEVEL

○ 1 ○ 2 ○ 3 ○ 4 ○ 5 ○ 6 ○ 7 ○ 8 ○ 9 ○ 10

MAIN INGREDIENTS

ADDITIONAL NOTES

WOULD YOU BUY IT AGAIN?		OVERALL RATING
○ YES	○ NO	/ 10

HOT SAUCE TASTING JOURNAL

NAME		BRAND	
ORIGIN		SAMPLED	
SCOVILLE		TEXTURE	
COLOR		PRICE	

HEAT

○ MEH	○ MILD
○ MEDIUM	○ HOT
○ VERY HOT	○ POWERFUL
○ PAINFUL	○ EXTREME

FLAVOR

○ LINGER	○ BERRY FRUIT	○ CITRUS FRUIT	○ TROPICAL FRUIT
○ DARK FRUIT	○ FLORAL	○ HERBAL	○ VEGETAL
○ GARLIC/ONION	○ VINEGAR	○ SALTY	○ SWEET
○ SPICES	○ SMOKY	○ ROASTY	○ CHOCOLATE

HEAT LEVEL

○ 1   ○ 2   ○ 3   ○ 4   ○ 5   ○ 6   ○ 7   ○ 8   ○ 9   ○ 10

MAIN INGREDIENTS

ADDITIONAL NOTES

WOULD YOU BUY IT AGAIN?	OVERALL RATING
○ YES ○ NO	/ 10

HOT SAUCE TASTING JOURNAL

NAME		BRAND	
ORIGIN		SAMPLED	
SCOVILLE		TEXTURE	
COLOR		PRICE	

HEAT	
○ MEH	○ MILD
○ MEDIUM	○ HOT
○ VERY HOT	○ POWERFUL
○ PAINFUL	○ EXTREME

FLAVOR			
○ LINGER	○ BERRY FRUIT	○ CITRUS FRUIT	○ TROPICAL FRUIT
○ DARK FRUIT	○ FLORAL	○ HERBAL	○ VEGETAL
○ GARLIC/ONION	○ VINEGAR	○ SALTY	○ SWEET
○ SPICES	○ SMOKY	○ ROASTY	○ CHOCOLATE

HEAT LEVEL

○ 1　○ 2　○ 3　○ 4　○ 5　○ 6　○ 7　○ 8　○ 9　○ 10

MAIN INGREDIENTS

_____
_____
_____
_____
_____
_____

ADDITIONAL NOTES

_____
_____
_____
_____

WOULD YOU BUY IT AGAIN?		OVERALL RATING
○ YES	○ NO	/ 10

HOT SAUCE TASTING JOURNAL

NAME		BRAND	
ORIGIN		SAMPLED	
SCOVILLE		TEXTURE	
COLOR		PRICE	

HEAT	
○ MEH	○ MILD
○ MEDIUM	○ HOT
○ VERY HOT	○ POWERFUL
○ PAINFUL	○ EXTREME

FLAVOR			
○ LINGER	○ BERRY FRUIT	○ CITRUS FRUIT	○ TROPICAL FRUIT
○ DARK FRUIT	○ FLORAL	○ HERBAL	○ VEGETAL
○ GARLIC/ONION	○ VINEGAR	○ SALTY	○ SWEET
○ SPICES	○ SMOKY	○ ROASTY	○ CHOCOLATE

HEAT LEVEL

○ 1 ○ 2 ○ 3 ○ 4 ○ 5 ○ 6 ○ 7 ○ 8 ○ 9 ○ 10

MAIN INGREDIENTS

ADDITIONAL NOTES

WOULD YOU BUY IT AGAIN?		OVERALL RATING
○ YES	○ NO	/ 10

HOT SAUCE TASTING JOURNAL

NAME		BRAND	
ORIGIN		SAMPLED	
SCOVILLE		TEXTURE	
COLOR		PRICE	

HEAT	
○ MEH	○ MILD
○ MEDIUM	○ HOT
○ VERY HOT	○ POWERFUL
○ PAINFUL	○ EXTREME

FLAVOR			
○ LINGER	○ BERRY FRUIT	○ CITRUS FRUIT	○ TROPICAL FRUIT
○ DARK FRUIT	○ FLORAL	○ HERBAL	○ VEGETAL
○ GARLIC/ONION	○ VINEGAR	○ SALTY	○ SWEET
○ SPICES	○ SMOKY	○ ROASTY	○ CHOCOLATE

HEAT LEVEL

○ 1 ○ 2 ○ 3 ○ 4 ○ 5 ○ 6 ○ 7 ○ 8 ○ 9 ○ 10

MAIN INGREDIENTS

ADDITIONAL NOTES

WOULD YOU BUY IT AGAIN?		OVERALL RATING
○ YES	○ NO	/ 10

HOT SAUCE TASTING JOURNAL

NAME		BRAND	
ORIGIN		SAMPLED	
SCOVILLE		TEXTURE	
COLOR		PRICE	

HEAT	
○ MEH	○ MILD
○ MEDIUM	○ HOT
○ VERY HOT	○ POWERFUL
○ PAINFUL	○ EXTREME

FLAVOR			
○ LINGER	○ BERRY FRUIT	○ CITRUS FRUIT	○ TROPICAL FRUIT
○ DARK FRUIT	○ FLORAL	○ HERBAL	○ VEGETAL
○ GARLIC/ONION	○ VINEGAR	○ SALTY	○ SWEET
○ SPICES	○ SMOKY	○ ROASTY	○ CHOCOLATE

HEAT LEVEL									
○ 1	○ 2	○ 3	○ 4	○ 5	○ 6	○ 7	○ 8	○ 9	○ 10

MAIN INGREDIENTS

ADDITIONAL NOTES

WOULD YOU BUY IT AGAIN?		OVERALL RATING
○ YES	○ NO	/ 10

HOT SAUCE TASTING JOURNAL

NAME		BRAND	
ORIGIN		SAMPLED	
SCOVILLE		TEXTURE	
COLOR		PRICE	

HEAT	
○ MEH	○ MILD
○ MEDIUM	○ HOT
○ VERY HOT	○ POWERFUL
○ PAINFUL	○ EXTREME

FLAVOR			
○ LINGER	○ BERRY FRUIT	○ CITRUS FRUIT	○ TROPICAL FRUIT
○ DARK FRUIT	○ FLORAL	○ HERBAL	○ VEGETAL
○ GARLIC/ONION	○ VINEGAR	○ SALTY	○ SWEET
○ SPICES	○ SMOKY	○ ROASTY	○ CHOCOLATE

HEAT LEVEL

○ 1   ○ 2   ○ 3   ○ 4   ○ 5   ○ 6   ○ 7   ○ 8   ○ 9   ○ 10

MAIN INGREDIENTS

ADDITIONAL NOTES

WOULD YOU BUY IT AGAIN?		OVERALL RATING
○ YES	○ NO	/ 10

HOT SAUCE TASTING JOURNAL

NAME		BRAND	
ORIGIN		SAMPLED	
SCOVILLE		TEXTURE	
COLOR		PRICE	

HEAT

○ MEH	○ MILD
○ MEDIUM	○ HOT
○ VERY HOT	○ POWERFUL
○ PAINFUL	○ EXTREME

FLAVOR

○ LINGER	○ BERRY FRUIT	○ CITRUS FRUIT	○ TROPICAL FRUIT
○ DARK FRUIT	○ FLORAL	○ HERBAL	○ VEGETAL
○ GARLIC/ONION	○ VINEGAR	○ SALTY	○ SWEET
○ SPICES	○ SMOKY	○ ROASTY	○ CHOCOLATE

HEAT LEVEL

○ 1　○ 2　○ 3　○ 4　○ 5　○ 6　○ 7　○ 8　○ 9　○ 10

MAIN INGREDIENTS

ADDITIONAL NOTES

WOULD YOU BUY IT AGAIN?		OVERALL RATING
○ YES	○ NO	/ 10

HOT SAUCE TASTING JOURNAL

NAME		BRAND	
ORIGIN		SAMPLED	
SCOVILLE		TEXTURE	
COLOR		PRICE	

HEAT

○ MEH	○ MILD
○ MEDIUM	○ HOT
○ VERY HOT	○ POWERFUL
○ PAINFUL	○ EXTREME

FLAVOR

○ LINGER	○ BERRY FRUIT	○ CITRUS FRUIT	○ TROPICAL FRUIT
○ DARK FRUIT	○ FLORAL	○ HERBAL	○ VEGETAL
○ GARLIC/ONION	○ VINEGAR	○ SALTY	○ SWEET
○ SPICES	○ SMOKY	○ ROASTY	○ CHOCOLATE

HEAT LEVEL

○ 1   ○ 2   ○ 3   ○ 4   ○ 5   ○ 6   ○ 7   ○ 8   ○ 9   ○ 10

MAIN INGREDIENTS

ADDITIONAL NOTES

WOULD YOU BUY IT AGAIN?		OVERALL RATING
○ YES	○ NO	/ 10

HOT SAUCE TASTING JOURNAL

NAME		BRAND	
ORIGIN		SAMPLED	
SCOVILLE		TEXTURE	
COLOR		PRICE	

HEAT

○ MEH	○ MILD
○ MEDIUM	○ HOT
○ VERY HOT	○ POWERFUL
○ PAINFUL	○ EXTREME

FLAVOR

○ LINGER	○ BERRY FRUIT	○ CITRUS FRUIT	○ TROPICAL FRUIT
○ DARK FRUIT	○ FLORAL	○ HERBAL	○ VEGETAL
○ GARLIC/ONION	○ VINEGAR	○ SALTY	○ SWEET
○ SPICES	○ SMOKY	○ ROASTY	○ CHOCOLATE

HEAT LEVEL

○ 1	○ 2	○ 3	○ 4	○ 5	○ 6	○ 7	○ 8	○ 9	○ 10

MAIN INGREDIENTS

ADDITIONAL NOTES

WOULD YOU BUY IT AGAIN?		OVERALL RATING
○ YES	○ NO	/ 10

HOT SAUCE TASTING JOURNAL

NAME		BRAND	
ORIGIN		SAMPLED	
SCOVILLE		TEXTURE	
COLOR		PRICE	

HEAT	
○ MEH	○ MILD
○ MEDIUM	○ HOT
○ VERY HOT	○ POWERFUL
○ PAINFUL	○ EXTREME

FLAVOR			
○ LINGER	○ BERRY FRUIT	○ CITRUS FRUIT	○ TROPICAL FRUIT
○ DARK FRUIT	○ FLORAL	○ HERBAL	○ VEGETAL
○ GARLIC/ONION	○ VINEGAR	○ SALTY	○ SWEET
○ SPICES	○ SMOKY	○ ROASTY	○ CHOCOLATE

HEAT LEVEL

○ 1 ○ 2 ○ 3 ○ 4 ○ 5 ○ 6 ○ 7 ○ 8 ○ 9 ○ 10

MAIN INGREDIENTS

ADDITIONAL NOTES

WOULD YOU BUY IT AGAIN?		OVERALL RATING
○ YES	○ NO	/ 10

HOT SAUCE TASTING JOURNAL

NAME		BRAND	
ORIGIN		SAMPLED	
SCOVILLE		TEXTURE	
COLOR		PRICE	

HEAT

○ MEH	○ MILD
○ MEDIUM	○ HOT
○ VERY HOT	○ POWERFUL
○ PAINFUL	○ EXTREME

FLAVOR

○ LINGER	○ BERRY FRUIT	○ CITRUS FRUIT	○ TROPICAL FRUIT
○ DARK FRUIT	○ FLORAL	○ HERBAL	○ VEGETAL
○ GARLIC/ONION	○ VINEGAR	○ SALTY	○ SWEET
○ SPICES	○ SMOKY	○ ROASTY	○ CHOCOLATE

HEAT LEVEL

○ 1	○ 2	○ 3	○ 4	○ 5	○ 6	○ 7	○ 8	○ 9	○ 10

MAIN INGREDIENTS

ADDITIONAL NOTES

WOULD YOU BUY IT AGAIN?		OVERALL RATING
○ YES	○ NO	/ 10

HOT SAUCE TASTING JOURNAL

NAME		BRAND	
ORIGIN		SAMPLED	
SCOVILLE		TEXTURE	
COLOR		PRICE	

HEAT	
○ MEH	○ MILD
○ MEDIUM	○ HOT
○ VERY HOT	○ POWERFUL
○ PAINFUL	○ EXTREME

FLAVOR			
○ LINGER	○ BERRY FRUIT	○ CITRUS FRUIT	○ TROPICAL FRUIT
○ DARK FRUIT	○ FLORAL	○ HERBAL	○ VEGETAL
○ GARLIC/ONION	○ VINEGAR	○ SALTY	○ SWEET
○ SPICES	○ SMOKY	○ ROASTY	○ CHOCOLATE

HEAT LEVEL

○ 1　○ 2　○ 3　○ 4　○ 5　○ 6　○ 7　○ 8　○ 9　○ 10

MAIN INGREDIENTS

ADDITIONAL NOTES

WOULD YOU BUY IT AGAIN?		OVERALL RATING
○ YES	○ NO	/ 10

HOT SAUCE TASTING JOURNAL

NAME		BRAND	
ORIGIN		SAMPLED	
SCOVILLE		TEXTURE	
COLOR		PRICE	

HEAT

○ MEH	○ MILD
○ MEDIUM	○ HOT
○ VERY HOT	○ POWERFUL
○ PAINFUL	○ EXTREME

FLAVOR

○ LINGER	○ BERRY FRUIT	○ CITRUS FRUIT	○ TROPICAL FRUIT
○ DARK FRUIT	○ FLORAL	○ HERBAL	○ VEGETAL
○ GARLIC/ONION	○ VINEGAR	○ SALTY	○ SWEET
○ SPICES	○ SMOKY	○ ROASTY	○ CHOCOLATE

HEAT LEVEL

○ 1   ○ 2   ○ 3   ○ 4   ○ 5   ○ 6   ○ 7   ○ 8   ○ 9   ○ 10

MAIN INGREDIENTS

ADDITIONAL NOTES

WOULD YOU BUY IT AGAIN?		OVERALL RATING
○ YES	○ NO	/ 10

HOT SAUCE TASTING JOURNAL

NAME		BRAND	
ORIGIN		SAMPLED	
SCOVILLE		TEXTURE	
COLOR		PRICE	

HEAT		FLAVOR			
○ MEH	○ MILD	○ LINGER	○ BERRY FRUIT	○ CITRUS FRUIT	○ TROPICAL FRUIT
○ MEDIUM	○ HOT	○ DARK FRUIT	○ FLORAL	○ HERBAL	○ VEGETAL
○ VERY HOT	○ POWERFUL	○ GARLIC/ONION	○ VINEGAR	○ SALTY	○ SWEET
○ PAINFUL	○ EXTREME	○ SPICES	○ SMOKY	○ ROASTY	○ CHOCOLATE

HEAT LEVEL

○ 1   ○ 2   ○ 3   ○ 4   ○ 5   ○ 6   ○ 7   ○ 8   ○ 9   ○ 10

MAIN INGREDIENTS

ADDITIONAL NOTES

WOULD YOU BUY IT AGAIN?		OVERALL RATING
○ YES	○ NO	/ 10

HOT SAUCE TASTING JOURNAL

NAME		BRAND	
ORIGIN		SAMPLED	
SCOVILLE		TEXTURE	
COLOR		PRICE	

HEAT	
○ MEH	○ MILD
○ MEDIUM	○ HOT
○ VERY HOT	○ POWERFUL
○ PAINFUL	○ EXTREME

FLAVOR			
○ LINGER	○ BERRY FRUIT	○ CITRUS FRUIT	○ TROPICAL FRUIT
○ DARK FRUIT	○ FLORAL	○ HERBAL	○ VEGETAL
○ GARLIC/ONION	○ VINEGAR	○ SALTY	○ SWEET
○ SPICES	○ SMOKY	○ ROASTY	○ CHOCOLATE

HEAT LEVEL									
○ 1	○ 2	○ 3	○ 4	○ 5	○ 6	○ 7	○ 8	○ 9	○ 10

MAIN INGREDIENTS

ADDITIONAL NOTES

WOULD YOU BUY IT AGAIN?		OVERALL RATING
○ YES	○ NO	/ 10

HOT SAUCE TASTING JOURNAL

NAME		BRAND	
ORIGIN		SAMPLED	
SCOVILLE		TEXTURE	
COLOR		PRICE	

HEAT	
○ MEH	○ MILD
○ MEDIUM	○ HOT
○ VERY HOT	○ POWERFUL
○ PAINFUL	○ EXTREME

FLAVOR			
○ LINGER	○ BERRY FRUIT	○ CITRUS FRUIT	○ TROPICAL FRUIT
○ DARK FRUIT	○ FLORAL	○ HERBAL	○ VEGETAL
○ GARLIC/ONION	○ VINEGAR	○ SALTY	○ SWEET
○ SPICES	○ SMOKY	○ ROASTY	○ CHOCOLATE

HEAT LEVEL

○ 1 ○ 2 ○ 3 ○ 4 ○ 5 ○ 6 ○ 7 ○ 8 ○ 9 ○ 10

MAIN INGREDIENTS

ADDITIONAL NOTES

WOULD YOU BUY IT AGAIN?		OVERALL RATING
○ YES	○ NO	/ 10

HOT SAUCE TASTING JOURNAL

NAME		BRAND	
ORIGIN		SAMPLED	
SCOVILLE		TEXTURE	
COLOR		PRICE	

HEAT

○ MEH	○ MILD
○ MEDIUM	○ HOT
○ VERY HOT	○ POWERFUL
○ PAINFUL	○ EXTREME

FLAVOR

○ LINGER	○ BERRY FRUIT	○ CITRUS FRUIT	○ TROPICAL FRUIT
○ DARK FRUIT	○ FLORAL	○ HERBAL	○ VEGETAL
○ GARLIC/ONION	○ VINEGAR	○ SALTY	○ SWEET
○ SPICES	○ SMOKY	○ ROASTY	○ CHOCOLATE

HEAT LEVEL

○ 1　○ 2　○ 3　○ 4　○ 5　○ 6　○ 7　○ 8　○ 9　○ 10

MAIN INGREDIENTS

ADDITIONAL NOTES

WOULD YOU BUY IT AGAIN?		OVERALL RATING
○ YES	○ NO	/ 10

HOT SAUCE TASTING JOURNAL

NAME		BRAND	
ORIGIN		SAMPLED	
SCOVILLE		TEXTURE	
COLOR		PRICE	

HEAT	
○ MEH	○ MILD
○ MEDIUM	○ HOT
○ VERY HOT	○ POWERFUL
○ PAINFUL	○ EXTREME

FLAVOR			
○ LINGER	○ BERRY FRUIT	○ CITRUS FRUIT	○ TROPICAL FRUIT
○ DARK FRUIT	○ FLORAL	○ HERBAL	○ VEGETAL
○ GARLIC/ONION	○ VINEGAR	○ SALTY	○ SWEET
○ SPICES	○ SMOKY	○ ROASTY	○ CHOCOLATE

HEAT LEVEL

○ 1 ○ 2 ○ 3 ○ 4 ○ 5 ○ 6 ○ 7 ○ 8 ○ 9 ○ 10

MAIN INGREDIENTS

ADDITIONAL NOTES

WOULD YOU BUY IT AGAIN?		OVERALL RATING
○ YES	○ NO	/ 10

HOT SAUCE TASTING JOURNAL

NAME		BRAND	
ORIGIN		SAMPLED	
SCOVILLE		TEXTURE	
COLOR		PRICE	

HEAT		FLAVOR			
○ MEH	○ MILD	○ LINGER	○ BERRY FRUIT	○ CITRUS FRUIT	○ TROPICAL FRUIT
○ MEDIUM	○ HOT	○ DARK FRUIT	○ FLORAL	○ HERBAL	○ VEGETAL
○ VERY HOT	○ POWERFUL	○ GARLIC/ONION	○ VINEGAR	○ SALTY	○ SWEET
○ PAINFUL	○ EXTREME	○ SPICES	○ SMOKY	○ ROASTY	○ CHOCOLATE

HEAT LEVEL									
○ 1	○ 2	○ 3	○ 4	○ 5	○ 6	○ 7	○ 8	○ 9	○ 10

MAIN INGREDIENTS

ADDITIONAL NOTES

WOULD YOU BUY IT AGAIN?		OVERALL RATING
○ YES	○ NO	/ 10

HOT SAUCE TASTING JOURNAL

NAME		BRAND	
ORIGIN		SAMPLED	
SCOVILLE		TEXTURE	
COLOR		PRICE	

HEAT

○ MEH	○ MILD
○ MEDIUM	○ HOT
○ VERY HOT	○ POWERFUL
○ PAINFUL	○ EXTREME

FLAVOR

○ LINGER	○ BERRY FRUIT	○ CITRUS FRUIT	○ TROPICAL FRUIT
○ DARK FRUIT	○ FLORAL	○ HERBAL	○ VEGETAL
○ GARLIC/ONION	○ VINEGAR	○ SALTY	○ SWEET
○ SPICES	○ SMOKY	○ ROASTY	○ CHOCOLATE

HEAT LEVEL

○ 1   ○ 2   ○ 3   ○ 4   ○ 5   ○ 6   ○ 7   ○ 8   ○ 9   ○ 10

MAIN INGREDIENTS

ADDITIONAL NOTES

WOULD YOU BUY IT AGAIN?		OVERALL RATING
○ YES	○ NO	/ 10

HOT SAUCE TASTING JOURNAL

NAME		BRAND	
ORIGIN		SAMPLED	
SCOVILLE		TEXTURE	
COLOR		PRICE	

HEAT		FLAVOR			
○ MEH	○ MILD	○ LINGER	○ BERRY FRUIT	○ CITRUS FRUIT	○ TROPICAL FRUIT
○ MEDIUM	○ HOT	○ DARK FRUIT	○ FLORAL	○ HERBAL	○ VEGETAL
○ VERY HOT	○ POWERFUL	○ GARLIC/ONION	○ VINEGAR	○ SALTY	○ SWEET
○ PAINFUL	○ EXTREME	○ SPICES	○ SMOKY	○ ROASTY	○ CHOCOLATE

HEAT LEVEL

○ 1 ○ 2 ○ 3 ○ 4 ○ 5 ○ 6 ○ 7 ○ 8 ○ 9 ○ 10

MAIN INGREDIENTS

ADDITIONAL NOTES

WOULD YOU BUY IT AGAIN?		OVERALL RATING
○ YES	○ NO	/ 10

HOT SAUCE TASTING JOURNAL

NAME		BRAND	
ORIGIN		SAMPLED	
SCOVILLE		TEXTURE	
COLOR		PRICE	

HEAT

○ MEH	○ MILD
○ MEDIUM	○ HOT
○ VERY HOT	○ POWERFUL
○ PAINFUL	○ EXTREME

FLAVOR

○ LINGER	○ BERRY FRUIT	○ CITRUS FRUIT	○ TROPICAL FRUIT
○ DARK FRUIT	○ FLORAL	○ HERBAL	○ VEGETAL
○ GARLIC/ONION	○ VINEGAR	○ SALTY	○ SWEET
○ SPICES	○ SMOKY	○ ROASTY	○ CHOCOLATE

HEAT LEVEL

○ 1 ○ 2 ○ 3 ○ 4 ○ 5 ○ 6 ○ 7 ○ 8 ○ 9 ○ 10

MAIN INGREDIENTS

ADDITIONAL NOTES

WOULD YOU BUY IT AGAIN?		OVERALL RATING
○ YES	○ NO	/ 10

HOT SAUCE TASTING JOURNAL

NAME		BRAND	
ORIGIN		SAMPLED	
SCOVILLE		TEXTURE	
COLOR		PRICE	

HEAT

○ MEH	○ MILD
○ MEDIUM	○ HOT
○ VERY HOT	○ POWERFUL
○ PAINFUL	○ EXTREME

FLAVOR

○ LINGER	○ BERRY FRUIT	○ CITRUS FRUIT	○ TROPICAL FRUIT
○ DARK FRUIT	○ FLORAL	○ HERBAL	○ VEGETAL
○ GARLIC/ONION	○ VINEGAR	○ SALTY	○ SWEET
○ SPICES	○ SMOKY	○ ROASTY	○ CHOCOLATE

HEAT LEVEL

○ 1	○ 2	○ 3	○ 4	○ 5	○ 6	○ 7	○ 8	○ 9	○ 10

MAIN INGREDIENTS

ADDITIONAL NOTES

WOULD YOU BUY IT AGAIN?		OVERALL RATING
○ YES	○ NO	/ 10

HOT SAUCE TASTING JOURNAL

NAME		BRAND	
ORIGIN		SAMPLED	
SCOVILLE		TEXTURE	
COLOR		PRICE	

HEAT			
○ MEH	○ MILD		
○ MEDIUM	○ HOT		
○ VERY HOT	○ POWERFUL		
○ PAINFUL	○ EXTREME		

FLAVOR			
○ LINGER	○ BERRY FRUIT	○ CITRUS FRUIT	○ TROPICAL FRUIT
○ DARK FRUIT	○ FLORAL	○ HERBAL	○ VEGETAL
○ GARLIC/ONION	○ VINEGAR	○ SALTY	○ SWEET
○ SPICES	○ SMOKY	○ ROASTY	○ CHOCOLATE

HEAT LEVEL

○ 1   ○ 2   ○ 3   ○ 4   ○ 5   ○ 6   ○ 7   ○ 8   ○ 9   ○ 10

MAIN INGREDIENTS

ADDITIONAL NOTES

WOULD YOU BUY IT AGAIN?		OVERALL RATING
○ YES	○ NO	/ 10

HOT SAUCE TASTING JOURNAL

NAME		BRAND	
ORIGIN		SAMPLED	
SCOVILLE		TEXTURE	
COLOR		PRICE	

HEAT	
○ MEH	○ MILD
○ MEDIUM	○ HOT
○ VERY HOT	○ POWERFUL
○ PAINFUL	○ EXTREME

FLAVOR			
○ LINGER	○ BERRY FRUIT	○ CITRUS FRUIT	○ TROPICAL FRUIT
○ DARK FRUIT	○ FLORAL	○ HERBAL	○ VEGETAL
○ GARLIC/ONION	○ VINEGAR	○ SALTY	○ SWEET
○ SPICES	○ SMOKY	○ ROASTY	○ CHOCOLATE

HEAT LEVEL									
○ 1	○ 2	○ 3	○ 4	○ 5	○ 6	○ 7	○ 8	○ 9	○ 10

MAIN INGREDIENTS

ADDITIONAL NOTES

WOULD YOU BUY IT AGAIN?		OVERALL RATING
○ YES	○ NO	/ 10

HOT SAUCE TASTING JOURNAL

NAME		BRAND	
ORIGIN		SAMPLED	
SCOVILLE		TEXTURE	
COLOR		PRICE	

HEAT	
○ MEH	○ MILD
○ MEDIUM	○ HOT
○ VERY HOT	○ POWERFUL
○ PAINFUL	○ EXTREME

FLAVOR			
○ LINGER	○ BERRY FRUIT	○ CITRUS FRUIT	○ TROPICAL FRUIT
○ DARK FRUIT	○ FLORAL	○ HERBAL	○ VEGETAL
○ GARLIC/ONION	○ VINEGAR	○ SALTY	○ SWEET
○ SPICES	○ SMOKY	○ ROASTY	○ CHOCOLATE

HEAT LEVEL									
○ 1	○ 2	○ 3	○ 4	○ 5	○ 6	○ 7	○ 8	○ 9	○ 10

MAIN INGREDIENTS

ADDITIONAL NOTES

WOULD YOU BUY IT AGAIN?		OVERALL RATING
○ YES	○ NO	/ 10

HOT SAUCE TASTING JOURNAL

NAME		BRAND	
ORIGIN		SAMPLED	
SCOVILLE		TEXTURE	
COLOR		PRICE	

HEAT	
○ MEH	○ MILD
○ MEDIUM	○ HOT
○ VERY HOT	○ POWERFUL
○ PAINFUL	○ EXTREME

FLAVOR			
○ LINGER	○ BERRY FRUIT	○ CITRUS FRUIT	○ TROPICAL FRUIT
○ DARK FRUIT	○ FLORAL	○ HERBAL	○ VEGETAL
○ GARLIC/ONION	○ VINEGAR	○ SALTY	○ SWEET
○ SPICES	○ SMOKY	○ ROASTY	○ CHOCOLATE

HEAT LEVEL									
○ 1	○ 2	○ 3	○ 4	○ 5	○ 6	○ 7	○ 8	○ 9	○ 10

MAIN INGREDIENTS

ADDITIONAL NOTES

WOULD YOU BUY IT AGAIN?		OVERALL RATING
○ YES	○ NO	/ 10

HOT SAUCE TASTING JOURNAL

NAME		BRAND	
ORIGIN		SAMPLED	
SCOVILLE		TEXTURE	
COLOR		PRICE	

HEAT	
○ MEH	○ MILD
○ MEDIUM	○ HOT
○ VERY HOT	○ POWERFUL
○ PAINFUL	○ EXTREME

FLAVOR			
○ LINGER	○ BERRY FRUIT	○ CITRUS FRUIT	○ TROPICAL FRUIT
○ DARK FRUIT	○ FLORAL	○ HERBAL	○ VEGETAL
○ GARLIC/ONION	○ VINEGAR	○ SALTY	○ SWEET
○ SPICES	○ SMOKY	○ ROASTY	○ CHOCOLATE

HEAT LEVEL

○ 1   ○ 2   ○ 3   ○ 4   ○ 5   ○ 6   ○ 7   ○ 8   ○ 9   ○ 10

MAIN INGREDIENTS

ADDITIONAL NOTES

WOULD YOU BUY IT AGAIN?		OVERALL RATING
○ YES	○ NO	/ 10

HOT SAUCE TASTING JOURNAL

NAME		BRAND	
ORIGIN		SAMPLED	
SCOVILLE		TEXTURE	
COLOR		PRICE	

HEAT	
○ MEH	○ MILD
○ MEDIUM	○ HOT
○ VERY HOT	○ POWERFUL
○ PAINFUL	○ EXTREME

FLAVOR			
○ LINGER	○ BERRY FRUIT	○ CITRUS FRUIT	○ TROPICAL FRUIT
○ DARK FRUIT	○ FLORAL	○ HERBAL	○ VEGETAL
○ GARLIC/ONION	○ VINEGAR	○ SALTY	○ SWEET
○ SPICES	○ SMOKY	○ ROASTY	○ CHOCOLATE

HEAT LEVEL

○ 1   ○ 2   ○ 3   ○ 4   ○ 5   ○ 6   ○ 7   ○ 8   ○ 9   ○ 10

MAIN INGREDIENTS

ADDITIONAL NOTES

WOULD YOU BUY IT AGAIN?		OVERALL RATING
○ YES	○ NO	/ 10

HOT SAUCE TASTING JOURNAL

NAME		BRAND	
ORIGIN		SAMPLED	
SCOVILLE		TEXTURE	
COLOR		PRICE	

HEAT		FLAVOR			
○ MEH	○ MILD	○ LINGER	○ BERRY FRUIT	○ CITRUS FRUIT	○ TROPICAL FRUIT
○ MEDIUM	○ HOT	○ DARK FRUIT	○ FLORAL	○ HERBAL	○ VEGETAL
○ VERY HOT	○ POWERFUL	○ GARLIC/ONION	○ VINEGAR	○ SALTY	○ SWEET
○ PAINFUL	○ EXTREME	○ SPICES	○ SMOKY	○ ROASTY	○ CHOCOLATE

HEAT LEVEL

○ 1	○ 2	○ 3	○ 4	○ 5	○ 6	○ 7	○ 8	○ 9	○ 10

MAIN INGREDIENTS

ADDITIONAL NOTES

WOULD YOU BUY IT AGAIN?		OVERALL RATING
○ YES	○ NO	/ 10

HOT SAUCE TASTING JOURNAL

NAME		BRAND	
ORIGIN		SAMPLED	
SCOVILLE		TEXTURE	
COLOR		PRICE	

HEAT		FLAVOR			
○ MEH	○ MILD	○ LINGER	○ BERRY FRUIT	○ CITRUS FRUIT	○ TROPICAL FRUIT
○ MEDIUM	○ HOT	○ DARK FRUIT	○ FLORAL	○ HERBAL	○ VEGETAL
○ VERY HOT	○ POWERFUL	○ GARLIC/ONION	○ VINEGAR	○ SALTY	○ SWEET
○ PAINFUL	○ EXTREME	○ SPICES	○ SMOKY	○ ROASTY	○ CHOCOLATE

HEAT LEVEL
○ 1 ○ 2 ○ 3 ○ 4 ○ 5 ○ 6 ○ 7 ○ 8 ○ 9 ○ 10

MAIN INGREDIENTS

ADDITIONAL NOTES

WOULD YOU BUY IT AGAIN?		OVERALL RATING
○ YES	○ NO	/ 10

HOT SAUCE TASTING JOURNAL

NAME		BRAND	
ORIGIN		SAMPLED	
SCOVILLE		TEXTURE	
COLOR		PRICE	

HEAT	
○ MEH	○ MILD
○ MEDIUM	○ HOT
○ VERY HOT	○ POWERFUL
○ PAINFUL	○ EXTREME

FLAVOR			
○ LINGER	○ BERRY FRUIT	○ CITRUS FRUIT	○ TROPICAL FRUIT
○ DARK FRUIT	○ FLORAL	○ HERBAL	○ VEGETAL
○ GARLIC/ONION	○ VINEGAR	○ SALTY	○ SWEET
○ SPICES	○ SMOKY	○ ROASTY	○ CHOCOLATE

HEAT LEVEL

○ 1 ○ 2 ○ 3 ○ 4 ○ 5 ○ 6 ○ 7 ○ 8 ○ 9 ○ 10

MAIN INGREDIENTS

ADDITIONAL NOTES

WOULD YOU BUY IT AGAIN?		OVERALL RATING
○ YES	○ NO	/ 10

HOT SAUCE TASTING JOURNAL

NAME		BRAND	
ORIGIN		SAMPLED	
SCOVILLE		TEXTURE	
COLOR		PRICE	

HEAT

○ MEH	○ MILD
○ MEDIUM	○ HOT
○ VERY HOT	○ POWERFUL
○ PAINFUL	○ EXTREME

FLAVOR

○ LINGER	○ BERRY FRUIT	○ CITRUS FRUIT	○ TROPICAL FRUIT
○ DARK FRUIT	○ FLORAL	○ HERBAL	○ VEGETAL
○ GARLIC/ONION	○ VINEGAR	○ SALTY	○ SWEET
○ SPICES	○ SMOKY	○ ROASTY	○ CHOCOLATE

HEAT LEVEL

○ 1	○ 2	○ 3	○ 4	○ 5	○ 6	○ 7	○ 8	○ 9	○ 10

MAIN INGREDIENTS

ADDITIONAL NOTES

WOULD YOU BUY IT AGAIN?		OVERALL RATING
○ YES	○ NO	/ 10

HOT SAUCE TASTING JOURNAL

NAME		BRAND	
ORIGIN		SAMPLED	
SCOVILLE		TEXTURE	
COLOR		PRICE	

HEAT		FLAVOR			
○ MEH	○ MILD	○ LINGER	○ BERRY FRUIT	○ CITRUS FRUIT	○ TROPICAL FRUIT
○ MEDIUM	○ HOT	○ DARK FRUIT	○ FLORAL	○ HERBAL	○ VEGETAL
○ VERY HOT	○ POWERFUL	○ GARLIC/ONION	○ VINEGAR	○ SALTY	○ SWEET
○ PAINFUL	○ EXTREME	○ SPICES	○ SMOKY	○ ROASTY	○ CHOCOLATE

HEAT LEVEL
○ 1　○ 2　○ 3　○ 4　○ 5　○ 6　○ 7　○ 8　○ 9　○ 10

MAIN INGREDIENTS

ADDITIONAL NOTES

WOULD YOU BUY IT AGAIN?		OVERALL RATING
○ YES	○ NO	/ 10

HOT SAUCE TASTING JOURNAL

NAME		BRAND	
ORIGIN		SAMPLED	
SCOVILLE		TEXTURE	
COLOR		PRICE	

HEAT	
○ MEH	○ MILD
○ MEDIUM	○ HOT
○ VERY HOT	○ POWERFUL
○ PAINFUL	○ EXTREME

FLAVOR			
○ LINGER	○ BERRY FRUIT	○ CITRUS FRUIT	○ TROPICAL FRUIT
○ DARK FRUIT	○ FLORAL	○ HERBAL	○ VEGETAL
○ GARLIC/ONION	○ VINEGAR	○ SALTY	○ SWEET
○ SPICES	○ SMOKY	○ ROASTY	○ CHOCOLATE

HEAT LEVEL

○ 1 ○ 2 ○ 3 ○ 4 ○ 5 ○ 6 ○ 7 ○ 8 ○ 9 ○ 10

MAIN INGREDIENTS

ADDITIONAL NOTES

WOULD YOU BUY IT AGAIN?		OVERALL RATING
○ YES	○ NO	/ 10

HOT SAUCE TASTING JOURNAL

NAME		BRAND	
ORIGIN		SAMPLED	
SCOVILLE		TEXTURE	
COLOR		PRICE	

HEAT

○ MEH	○ MILD
○ MEDIUM	○ HOT
○ VERY HOT	○ POWERFUL
○ PAINFUL	○ EXTREME

FLAVOR

○ LINGER	○ BERRY FRUIT	○ CITRUS FRUIT	○ TROPICAL FRUIT
○ DARK FRUIT	○ FLORAL	○ HERBAL	○ VEGETAL
○ GARLIC/ONION	○ VINEGAR	○ SALTY	○ SWEET
○ SPICES	○ SMOKY	○ ROASTY	○ CHOCOLATE

HEAT LEVEL

○ 1 ○ 2 ○ 3 ○ 4 ○ 5 ○ 6 ○ 7 ○ 8 ○ 9 ○ 10

MAIN INGREDIENTS

ADDITIONAL NOTES

WOULD YOU BUY IT AGAIN?		OVERALL RATING
○ YES	○ NO	/ 10

HOT SAUCE TASTING JOURNAL

NAME		BRAND	
ORIGIN		SAMPLED	
SCOVILLE		TEXTURE	
COLOR		PRICE	

HEAT

○ MEH	○ MILD
○ MEDIUM	○ HOT
○ VERY HOT	○ POWERFUL
○ PAINFUL	○ EXTREME

FLAVOR

○ LINGER	○ BERRY FRUIT	○ CITRUS FRUIT	○ TROPICAL FRUIT
○ DARK FRUIT	○ FLORAL	○ HERBAL	○ VEGETAL
○ GARLIC/ONION	○ VINEGAR	○ SALTY	○ SWEET
○ SPICES	○ SMOKY	○ ROASTY	○ CHOCOLATE

HEAT LEVEL

○ 1	○ 2	○ 3	○ 4	○ 5	○ 6	○ 7	○ 8	○ 9	○ 10

MAIN INGREDIENTS

ADDITIONAL NOTES

WOULD YOU BUY IT AGAIN?		OVERALL RATING
○ YES	○ NO	/ 10

HOT SAUCE TASTING JOURNAL

NAME		BRAND	
ORIGIN		SAMPLED	
SCOVILLE		TEXTURE	
COLOR		PRICE	

HEAT	
○ MEH	○ MILD
○ MEDIUM	○ HOT
○ VERY HOT	○ POWERFUL
○ PAINFUL	○ EXTREME

FLAVOR			
○ LINGER	○ BERRY FRUIT	○ CITRUS FRUIT	○ TROPICAL FRUIT
○ DARK FRUIT	○ FLORAL	○ HERBAL	○ VEGETAL
○ GARLIC/ONION	○ VINEGAR	○ SALTY	○ SWEET
○ SPICES	○ SMOKY	○ ROASTY	○ CHOCOLATE

HEAT LEVEL									
○ 1	○ 2	○ 3	○ 4	○ 5	○ 6	○ 7	○ 8	○ 9	○ 10

MAIN INGREDIENTS

ADDITIONAL NOTES

WOULD YOU BUY IT AGAIN?		OVERALL RATING
○ YES	○ NO	/ 10

HOT SAUCE TASTING JOURNAL

NAME		BRAND	
ORIGIN		SAMPLED	
SCOVILLE		TEXTURE	
COLOR		PRICE	

HEAT

○ MEH	○ MILD
○ MEDIUM	○ HOT
○ VERY HOT	○ POWERFUL
○ PAINFUL	○ EXTREME

FLAVOR

○ LINGER	○ BERRY FRUIT	○ CITRUS FRUIT	○ TROPICAL FRUIT
○ DARK FRUIT	○ FLORAL	○ HERBAL	○ VEGETAL
○ GARLIC/ONION	○ VINEGAR	○ SALTY	○ SWEET
○ SPICES	○ SMOKY	○ ROASTY	○ CHOCOLATE

HEAT LEVEL

○ 1 ○ 2 ○ 3 ○ 4 ○ 5 ○ 6 ○ 7 ○ 8 ○ 9 ○ 10

MAIN INGREDIENTS

_____
_____
_____
_____
_____
_____

ADDITIONAL NOTES

_____
_____
_____
_____
_____

WOULD YOU BUY IT AGAIN?		OVERALL RATING
○ YES	○ NO	/ 10

HOT SAUCE TASTING JOURNAL

NAME		BRAND	
ORIGIN		SAMPLED	
SCOVILLE		TEXTURE	
COLOR		PRICE	

HEAT	
○ MEH	○ MILD
○ MEDIUM	○ HOT
○ VERY HOT	○ POWERFUL
○ PAINFUL	○ EXTREME

FLAVOR			
○ LINGER	○ BERRY FRUIT	○ CITRUS FRUIT	○ TROPICAL FRUIT
○ DARK FRUIT	○ FLORAL	○ HERBAL	○ VEGETAL
○ GARLIC/ONION	○ VINEGAR	○ SALTY	○ SWEET
○ SPICES	○ SMOKY	○ ROASTY	○ CHOCOLATE

HEAT LEVEL

○ 1 ○ 2 ○ 3 ○ 4 ○ 5 ○ 6 ○ 7 ○ 8 ○ 9 ○ 10

MAIN INGREDIENTS

ADDITIONAL NOTES

WOULD YOU BUY IT AGAIN?		OVERALL RATING
○ YES	○ NO	/ 10

HOT SAUCE TASTING JOURNAL

NAME		BRAND	
ORIGIN		SAMPLED	
SCOVILLE		TEXTURE	
COLOR		PRICE	

HEAT

○ MEH	○ MILD
○ MEDIUM	○ HOT
○ VERY HOT	○ POWERFUL
○ PAINFUL	○ EXTREME

FLAVOR

○ LINGER	○ BERRY FRUIT	○ CITRUS FRUIT	○ TROPICAL FRUIT
○ DARK FRUIT	○ FLORAL	○ HERBAL	○ VEGETAL
○ GARLIC/ONION	○ VINEGAR	○ SALTY	○ SWEET
○ SPICES	○ SMOKY	○ ROASTY	○ CHOCOLATE

HEAT LEVEL

○ 1　○ 2　○ 3　○ 4　○ 5　○ 6　○ 7　○ 8　○ 9　○ 10

MAIN INGREDIENTS

ADDITIONAL NOTES

WOULD YOU BUY IT AGAIN?		OVERALL RATING
○ YES	○ NO	/ 10

HOT SAUCE TASTING JOURNAL

NAME		BRAND	
ORIGIN		SAMPLED	
SCOVILLE		TEXTURE	
COLOR		PRICE	

HEAT		FLAVOR			
○ MEH	○ MILD	○ LINGER	○ BERRY FRUIT	○ CITRUS FRUIT	○ TROPICAL FRUIT
○ MEDIUM	○ HOT	○ DARK FRUIT	○ FLORAL	○ HERBAL	○ VEGETAL
○ VERY HOT	○ POWERFUL	○ GARLIC/ONION	○ VINEGAR	○ SALTY	○ SWEET
○ PAINFUL	○ EXTREME	○ SPICES	○ SMOKY	○ ROASTY	○ CHOCOLATE

HEAT LEVEL

○ 1　○ 2　○ 3　○ 4　○ 5　○ 6　○ 7　○ 8　○ 9　○ 10

MAIN INGREDIENTS

ADDITIONAL NOTES

WOULD YOU BUY IT AGAIN?		OVERALL RATING
○ YES	○ NO	/ 10

HOT SAUCE TASTING JOURNAL

NAME		BRAND	
ORIGIN		SAMPLED	
SCOVILLE		TEXTURE	
COLOR		PRICE	

HEAT

○ MEH	○ MILD
○ MEDIUM	○ HOT
○ VERY HOT	○ POWERFUL
○ PAINFUL	○ EXTREME

FLAVOR

○ LINGER	○ BERRY FRUIT	○ CITRUS FRUIT	○ TROPICAL FRUIT
○ DARK FRUIT	○ FLORAL	○ HERBAL	○ VEGETAL
○ GARLIC/ONION	○ VINEGAR	○ SALTY	○ SWEET
○ SPICES	○ SMOKY	○ ROASTY	○ CHOCOLATE

HEAT LEVEL

○ 1　○ 2　○ 3　○ 4　○ 5　○ 6　○ 7　○ 8　○ 9　○ 10

MAIN INGREDIENTS

ADDITIONAL NOTES

WOULD YOU BUY IT AGAIN?		OVERALL RATING
○ YES	○ NO	/ 10

HOT SAUCE TASTING JOURNAL

NAME		BRAND	
ORIGIN		SAMPLED	
SCOVILLE		TEXTURE	
COLOR		PRICE	

HEAT

○ MEH	○ MILD
○ MEDIUM	○ HOT
○ VERY HOT	○ POWERFUL
○ PAINFUL	○ EXTREME

FLAVOR

○ LINGER	○ BERRY FRUIT	○ CITRUS FRUIT	○ TROPICAL FRUIT
○ DARK FRUIT	○ FLORAL	○ HERBAL	○ VEGETAL
○ GARLIC/ONION	○ VINEGAR	○ SALTY	○ SWEET
○ SPICES	○ SMOKY	○ ROASTY	○ CHOCOLATE

HEAT LEVEL

○ 1　○ 2　○ 3　○ 4　○ 5　○ 6　○ 7　○ 8　○ 9　○ 10

MAIN INGREDIENTS

ADDITIONAL NOTES

WOULD YOU BUY IT AGAIN?		OVERALL RATING
○ YES	○ NO	/ 10

HOT SAUCE TASTING JOURNAL

NAME		BRAND	
ORIGIN		SAMPLED	
SCOVILLE		TEXTURE	
COLOR		PRICE	

HEAT

○ MEH	○ MILD
○ MEDIUM	○ HOT
○ VERY HOT	○ POWERFUL
○ PAINFUL	○ EXTREME

FLAVOR

○ LINGER	○ BERRY FRUIT	○ CITRUS FRUIT	○ TROPICAL FRUIT
○ DARK FRUIT	○ FLORAL	○ HERBAL	○ VEGETAL
○ GARLIC/ONION	○ VINEGAR	○ SALTY	○ SWEET
○ SPICES	○ SMOKY	○ ROASTY	○ CHOCOLATE

HEAT LEVEL

○ 1　○ 2　○ 3　○ 4　○ 5　○ 6　○ 7　○ 8　○ 9　○ 10

MAIN INGREDIENTS

_____
_____
_____
_____
_____
_____

ADDITIONAL NOTES

_____
_____
_____
_____

WOULD YOU BUY IT AGAIN?		OVERALL RATING
○ YES	○ NO	/ 10

HOT SAUCE TASTING JOURNAL

NAME		BRAND	
ORIGIN		SAMPLED	
SCOVILLE		TEXTURE	
COLOR		PRICE	

HEAT

○ MEH	○ MILD
○ MEDIUM	○ HOT
○ VERY HOT	○ POWERFUL
○ PAINFUL	○ EXTREME

FLAVOR

○ LINGER	○ BERRY FRUIT	○ CITRUS FRUIT	○ TROPICAL FRUIT
○ DARK FRUIT	○ FLORAL	○ HERBAL	○ VEGETAL
○ GARLIC/ONION	○ VINEGAR	○ SALTY	○ SWEET
○ SPICES	○ SMOKY	○ ROASTY	○ CHOCOLATE

HEAT LEVEL

○ 1   ○ 2   ○ 3   ○ 4   ○ 5   ○ 6   ○ 7   ○ 8   ○ 9   ○ 10

MAIN INGREDIENTS

ADDITIONAL NOTES

WOULD YOU BUY IT AGAIN?		OVERALL RATING
○ YES	○ NO	/ 10

HOT SAUCE TASTING JOURNAL

NAME		BRAND	
ORIGIN		SAMPLED	
SCOVILLE		TEXTURE	
COLOR		PRICE	

HEAT

○ MEH	○ MILD
○ MEDIUM	○ HOT
○ VERY HOT	○ POWERFUL
○ PAINFUL	○ EXTREME

FLAVOR

○ LINGER	○ BERRY FRUIT	○ CITRUS FRUIT	○ TROPICAL FRUIT
○ DARK FRUIT	○ FLORAL	○ HERBAL	○ VEGETAL
○ GARLIC/ONION	○ VINEGAR	○ SALTY	○ SWEET
○ SPICES	○ SMOKY	○ ROASTY	○ CHOCOLATE

HEAT LEVEL

○ 1   ○ 2   ○ 3   ○ 4   ○ 5   ○ 6   ○ 7   ○ 8   ○ 9   ○ 10

MAIN INGREDIENTS

ADDITIONAL NOTES

WOULD YOU BUY IT AGAIN?		OVERALL RATING
○ YES	○ NO	/ 10

HOT SAUCE TASTING JOURNAL

NAME		BRAND	
ORIGIN		SAMPLED	
SCOVILLE		TEXTURE	
COLOR		PRICE	

HEAT

○ MEH	○ MILD
○ MEDIUM	○ HOT
○ VERY HOT	○ POWERFUL
○ PAINFUL	○ EXTREME

FLAVOR

○ LINGER	○ BERRY FRUIT	○ CITRUS FRUIT	○ TROPICAL FRUIT
○ DARK FRUIT	○ FLORAL	○ HERBAL	○ VEGETAL
○ GARLIC/ONION	○ VINEGAR	○ SALTY	○ SWEET
○ SPICES	○ SMOKY	○ ROASTY	○ CHOCOLATE

HEAT LEVEL

○ 1 ○ 2 ○ 3 ○ 4 ○ 5 ○ 6 ○ 7 ○ 8 ○ 9 ○ 10

MAIN INGREDIENTS

ADDITIONAL NOTES

WOULD YOU BUY IT AGAIN?		OVERALL RATING
○ YES	○ NO	/ 10

HOT SAUCE TASTING JOURNAL

NAME		BRAND	
ORIGIN		SAMPLED	
SCOVILLE		TEXTURE	
COLOR		PRICE	

HEAT	
○ MEH	○ MILD
○ MEDIUM	○ HOT
○ VERY HOT	○ POWERFUL
○ PAINFUL	○ EXTREME

FLAVOR			
○ LINGER	○ BERRY FRUIT	○ CITRUS FRUIT	○ TROPICAL FRUIT
○ DARK FRUIT	○ FLORAL	○ HERBAL	○ VEGETAL
○ GARLIC/ONION	○ VINEGAR	○ SALTY	○ SWEET
○ SPICES	○ SMOKY	○ ROASTY	○ CHOCOLATE

HEAT LEVEL

○ 1   ○ 2   ○ 3   ○ 4   ○ 5   ○ 6   ○ 7   ○ 8   ○ 9   ○ 10

MAIN INGREDIENTS

ADDITIONAL NOTES

WOULD YOU BUY IT AGAIN?		OVERALL RATING
○ YES	○ NO	/ 10

HOT SAUCE TASTING JOURNAL

NAME		BRAND	
ORIGIN		SAMPLED	
SCOVILLE		TEXTURE	
COLOR		PRICE	

HEAT

○ MEH	○ MILD
○ MEDIUM	○ HOT
○ VERY HOT	○ POWERFUL
○ PAINFUL	○ EXTREME

FLAVOR

○ LINGER	○ BERRY FRUIT	○ CITRUS FRUIT	○ TROPICAL FRUIT
○ DARK FRUIT	○ FLORAL	○ HERBAL	○ VEGETAL
○ GARLIC/ONION	○ VINEGAR	○ SALTY	○ SWEET
○ SPICES	○ SMOKY	○ ROASTY	○ CHOCOLATE

HEAT LEVEL

○ 1   ○ 2   ○ 3   ○ 4   ○ 5   ○ 6   ○ 7   ○ 8   ○ 9   ○ 10

MAIN INGREDIENTS

ADDITIONAL NOTES

WOULD YOU BUY IT AGAIN?		OVERALL RATING
○ YES	○ NO	/ 10

HOT SAUCE TASTING JOURNAL

NAME		BRAND	
ORIGIN		SAMPLED	
SCOVILLE		TEXTURE	
COLOR		PRICE	

HEAT

○ MEH	○ MILD
○ MEDIUM	○ HOT
○ VERY HOT	○ POWERFUL
○ PAINFUL	○ EXTREME

FLAVOR

○ LINGER	○ BERRY FRUIT	○ CITRUS FRUIT	○ TROPICAL FRUIT
○ DARK FRUIT	○ FLORAL	○ HERBAL	○ VEGETAL
○ GARLIC/ONION	○ VINEGAR	○ SALTY	○ SWEET
○ SPICES	○ SMOKY	○ ROASTY	○ CHOCOLATE

HEAT LEVEL

○ 1	○ 2	○ 3	○ 4	○ 5	○ 6	○ 7	○ 8	○ 9	○ 10

MAIN INGREDIENTS

ADDITIONAL NOTES

WOULD YOU BUY IT AGAIN?		OVERALL RATING
○ YES	○ NO	/ 10

HOT SAUCE TASTING JOURNAL

NAME		BRAND	
ORIGIN		SAMPLED	
SCOVILLE		TEXTURE	
COLOR		PRICE	

HEAT	
○ MEH	○ MILD
○ MEDIUM	○ HOT
○ VERY HOT	○ POWERFUL
○ PAINFUL	○ EXTREME

FLAVOR			
○ LINGER	○ BERRY FRUIT	○ CITRUS FRUIT	○ TROPICAL FRUIT
○ DARK FRUIT	○ FLORAL	○ HERBAL	○ VEGETAL
○ GARLIC/ONION	○ VINEGAR	○ SALTY	○ SWEET
○ SPICES	○ SMOKY	○ ROASTY	○ CHOCOLATE

HEAT LEVEL

○ 1 ○ 2 ○ 3 ○ 4 ○ 5 ○ 6 ○ 7 ○ 8 ○ 9 ○ 10

MAIN INGREDIENTS

ADDITIONAL NOTES

WOULD YOU BUY IT AGAIN?		OVERALL RATING
○ YES	○ NO	/ 10

HOT SAUCE TASTING JOURNAL

NAME		BRAND	
ORIGIN		SAMPLED	
SCOVILLE		TEXTURE	
COLOR		PRICE	

HEAT	
○ MEH	○ MILD
○ MEDIUM	○ HOT
○ VERY HOT	○ POWERFUL
○ PAINFUL	○ EXTREME

FLAVOR			
○ LINGER	○ BERRY FRUIT	○ CITRUS FRUIT	○ TROPICAL FRUIT
○ DARK FRUIT	○ FLORAL	○ HERBAL	○ VEGETAL
○ GARLIC/ONION	○ VINEGAR	○ SALTY	○ SWEET
○ SPICES	○ SMOKY	○ ROASTY	○ CHOCOLATE

HEAT LEVEL									
○ 1	○ 2	○ 3	○ 4	○ 5	○ 6	○ 7	○ 8	○ 9	○ 10

MAIN INGREDIENTS

ADDITIONAL NOTES

WOULD YOU BUY IT AGAIN?		OVERALL RATING
○ YES	○ NO	/ 10

HOT SAUCE TASTING JOURNAL

NAME		BRAND	
ORIGIN		SAMPLED	
SCOVILLE		TEXTURE	
COLOR		PRICE	

HEAT	
○ MEH	○ MILD
○ MEDIUM	○ HOT
○ VERY HOT	○ POWERFUL
○ PAINFUL	○ EXTREME

FLAVOR			
○ LINGER	○ BERRY FRUIT	○ CITRUS FRUIT	○ TROPICAL FRUIT
○ DARK FRUIT	○ FLORAL	○ HERBAL	○ VEGETAL
○ GARLIC/ONION	○ VINEGAR	○ SALTY	○ SWEET
○ SPICES	○ SMOKY	○ ROASTY	○ CHOCOLATE

HEAT LEVEL

○ 1 ○ 2 ○ 3 ○ 4 ○ 5 ○ 6 ○ 7 ○ 8 ○ 9 ○ 10

MAIN INGREDIENTS

ADDITIONAL NOTES

WOULD YOU BUY IT AGAIN?		OVERALL RATING
○ YES	○ NO	/ 10

HOT SAUCE TASTING JOURNAL

NAME		BRAND	
ORIGIN		SAMPLED	
SCOVILLE		TEXTURE	
COLOR		PRICE	

HEAT	
○ MEH	○ MILD
○ MEDIUM	○ HOT
○ VERY HOT	○ POWERFUL
○ PAINFUL	○ EXTREME

FLAVOR			
○ LINGER	○ BERRY FRUIT	○ CITRUS FRUIT	○ TROPICAL FRUIT
○ DARK FRUIT	○ FLORAL	○ HERBAL	○ VEGETAL
○ GARLIC/ONION	○ VINEGAR	○ SALTY	○ SWEET
○ SPICES	○ SMOKY	○ ROASTY	○ CHOCOLATE

HEAT LEVEL									
○ 1	○ 2	○ 3	○ 4	○ 5	○ 6	○ 7	○ 8	○ 9	○ 10

MAIN INGREDIENTS

ADDITIONAL NOTES

WOULD YOU BUY IT AGAIN?		OVERALL RATING
○ YES	○ NO	/ 10

HOT SAUCE TASTING JOURNAL

NAME		BRAND	
ORIGIN		SAMPLED	
SCOVILLE		TEXTURE	
COLOR		PRICE	

HEAT	
○ MEH	○ MILD
○ MEDIUM	○ HOT
○ VERY HOT	○ POWERFUL
○ PAINFUL	○ EXTREME

FLAVOR			
○ LINGER	○ BERRY FRUIT	○ CITRUS FRUIT	○ TROPICAL FRUIT
○ DARK FRUIT	○ FLORAL	○ HERBAL	○ VEGETAL
○ GARLIC/ONION	○ VINEGAR	○ SALTY	○ SWEET
○ SPICES	○ SMOKY	○ ROASTY	○ CHOCOLATE

HEAT LEVEL
○ 1　○ 2　○ 3　○ 4　○ 5　○ 6　○ 7　○ 8　○ 9　○ 10

MAIN INGREDIENTS

ADDITIONAL NOTES

WOULD YOU BUY IT AGAIN?		OVERALL RATING
○ YES	○ NO	/ 10

HOT SAUCE TASTING JOURNAL

NAME		BRAND	
ORIGIN		SAMPLED	
SCOVILLE		TEXTURE	
COLOR		PRICE	

HEAT			FLAVOR			
○ MEH	○ MILD		○ LINGER	○ BERRY FRUIT	○ CITRUS FRUIT	○ TROPICAL FRUIT
○ MEDIUM	○ HOT		○ DARK FRUIT	○ FLORAL	○ HERBAL	○ VEGETAL
○ VERY HOT	○ POWERFUL		○ GARLIC/ONION	○ VINEGAR	○ SALTY	○ SWEET
○ PAINFUL	○ EXTREME		○ SPICES	○ SMOKY	○ ROASTY	○ CHOCOLATE

HEAT LEVEL

○ 1　　○ 2　　○ 3　　○ 4　　○ 5　　○ 6　　○ 7　　○ 8　　○ 9　　○ 10

MAIN INGREDIENTS

ADDITIONAL NOTES

WOULD YOU BUY IT AGAIN?		OVERALL RATING
○ YES	○ NO	/ 10

HOT SAUCE TASTING JOURNAL

NAME		BRAND	
ORIGIN		SAMPLED	
SCOVILLE		TEXTURE	
COLOR		PRICE	

HEAT	
○ MEH	○ MILD
○ MEDIUM	○ HOT
○ VERY HOT	○ POWERFUL
○ PAINFUL	○ EXTREME

FLAVOR			
○ LINGER	○ BERRY FRUIT	○ CITRUS FRUIT	○ TROPICAL FRUIT
○ DARK FRUIT	○ FLORAL	○ HERBAL	○ VEGETAL
○ GARLIC/ONION	○ VINEGAR	○ SALTY	○ SWEET
○ SPICES	○ SMOKY	○ ROASTY	○ CHOCOLATE

HEAT LEVEL

○ 1 | ○ 2 | ○ 3 | ○ 4 | ○ 5 | ○ 6 | ○ 7 | ○ 8 | ○ 9 | ○ 10

MAIN INGREDIENTS

ADDITIONAL NOTES

WOULD YOU BUY IT AGAIN?		OVERALL RATING
○ YES	○ NO	/ 10

HOT SAUCE TASTING JOURNAL

NAME		BRAND	
ORIGIN		SAMPLED	
SCOVILLE		TEXTURE	
COLOR		PRICE	

HEAT

○ MEH	○ MILD		
○ MEDIUM	○ HOT		
○ VERY HOT	○ POWERFUL		
○ PAINFUL	○ EXTREME		

FLAVOR

○ LINGER	○ BERRY FRUIT	○ CITRUS FRUIT	○ TROPICAL FRUIT
○ DARK FRUIT	○ FLORAL	○ HERBAL	○ VEGETAL
○ GARLIC/ONION	○ VINEGAR	○ SALTY	○ SWEET
○ SPICES	○ SMOKY	○ ROASTY	○ CHOCOLATE

HEAT LEVEL

○ 1	○ 2	○ 3	○ 4	○ 5	○ 6	○ 7	○ 8	○ 9	○ 10

MAIN INGREDIENTS

ADDITIONAL NOTES

WOULD YOU BUY IT AGAIN?		OVERALL RATING
○ YES	○ NO	/ 10

HOT SAUCE TASTING JOURNAL

NAME		BRAND	
ORIGIN		SAMPLED	
SCOVILLE		TEXTURE	
COLOR		PRICE	

HEAT	
○ MEH	○ MILD
○ MEDIUM	○ HOT
○ VERY HOT	○ POWERFUL
○ PAINFUL	○ EXTREME

FLAVOR			
○ LINGER	○ BERRY FRUIT	○ CITRUS FRUIT	○ TROPICAL FRUIT
○ DARK FRUIT	○ FLORAL	○ HERBAL	○ VEGETAL
○ GARLIC/ONION	○ VINEGAR	○ SALTY	○ SWEET
○ SPICES	○ SMOKY	○ ROASTY	○ CHOCOLATE

HEAT LEVEL									
○ 1	○ 2	○ 3	○ 4	○ 5	○ 6	○ 7	○ 8	○ 9	○ 10

MAIN INGREDIENTS

ADDITIONAL NOTES

WOULD YOU BUY IT AGAIN?		OVERALL RATING
○ YES	○ NO	/ 10

HOT SAUCE TASTING JOURNAL

NAME		BRAND	
ORIGIN		SAMPLED	
SCOVILLE		TEXTURE	
COLOR		PRICE	

HEAT	
○ MEH	○ MILD
○ MEDIUM	○ HOT
○ VERY HOT	○ POWERFUL
○ PAINFUL	○ EXTREME

FLAVOR			
○ LINGER	○ BERRY FRUIT	○ CITRUS FRUIT	○ TROPICAL FRUIT
○ DARK FRUIT	○ FLORAL	○ HERBAL	○ VEGETAL
○ GARLIC/ONION	○ VINEGAR	○ SALTY	○ SWEET
○ SPICES	○ SMOKY	○ ROASTY	○ CHOCOLATE

HEAT LEVEL									
○ 1	○ 2	○ 3	○ 4	○ 5	○ 6	○ 7	○ 8	○ 9	○ 10

MAIN INGREDIENTS

ADDITIONAL NOTES

WOULD YOU BUY IT AGAIN?		OVERALL RATING
○ YES	○ NO	/ 10

HOT SAUCE TASTING JOURNAL

NAME		BRAND	
ORIGIN		SAMPLED	
SCOVILLE		TEXTURE	
COLOR		PRICE	

HEAT	
○ MEH	○ MILD
○ MEDIUM	○ HOT
○ VERY HOT	○ POWERFUL
○ PAINFUL	○ EXTREME

FLAVOR			
○ LINGER	○ BERRY FRUIT	○ CITRUS FRUIT	○ TROPICAL FRUIT
○ DARK FRUIT	○ FLORAL	○ HERBAL	○ VEGETAL
○ GARLIC/ONION	○ VINEGAR	○ SALTY	○ SWEET
○ SPICES	○ SMOKY	○ ROASTY	○ CHOCOLATE

HEAT LEVEL									
○ 1	○ 2	○ 3	○ 4	○ 5	○ 6	○ 7	○ 8	○ 9	○ 10

MAIN INGREDIENTS

ADDITIONAL NOTES

WOULD YOU BUY IT AGAIN?		OVERALL RATING
○ YES	○ NO	/ 10

HOT SAUCE TASTING JOURNAL

NAME		BRAND	
ORIGIN		SAMPLED	
SCOVILLE		TEXTURE	
COLOR		PRICE	

HEAT

○ MEH	○ MILD
○ MEDIUM	○ HOT
○ VERY HOT	○ POWERFUL
○ PAINFUL	○ EXTREME

FLAVOR

○ LINGER	○ BERRY FRUIT	○ CITRUS FRUIT	○ TROPICAL FRUIT
○ DARK FRUIT	○ FLORAL	○ HERBAL	○ VEGETAL
○ GARLIC/ONION	○ VINEGAR	○ SALTY	○ SWEET
○ SPICES	○ SMOKY	○ ROASTY	○ CHOCOLATE

HEAT LEVEL

○ 1 ○ 2 ○ 3 ○ 4 ○ 5 ○ 6 ○ 7 ○ 8 ○ 9 ○ 10

MAIN INGREDIENTS

ADDITIONAL NOTES

WOULD YOU BUY IT AGAIN?		OVERALL RATING
○ YES	○ NO	/ 10

HOT SAUCE TASTING JOURNAL

NAME		BRAND	
ORIGIN		SAMPLED	
SCOVILLE		TEXTURE	
COLOR		PRICE	

HEAT	
○ MEH	○ MILD
○ MEDIUM	○ HOT
○ VERY HOT	○ POWERFUL
○ PAINFUL	○ EXTREME

FLAVOR			
○ LINGER	○ BERRY FRUIT	○ CITRUS FRUIT	○ TROPICAL FRUIT
○ DARK FRUIT	○ FLORAL	○ HERBAL	○ VEGETAL
○ GARLIC/ONION	○ VINEGAR	○ SALTY	○ SWEET
○ SPICES	○ SMOKY	○ ROASTY	○ CHOCOLATE

HEAT LEVEL

○ 1   ○ 2   ○ 3   ○ 4   ○ 5   ○ 6   ○ 7   ○ 8   ○ 9   ○ 10

MAIN INGREDIENTS

ADDITIONAL NOTES

WOULD YOU BUY IT AGAIN?		OVERALL RATING
○ YES	○ NO	/ 10

HOT SAUCE TASTING JOURNAL

NAME		BRAND	
ORIGIN		SAMPLED	
SCOVILLE		TEXTURE	
COLOR		PRICE	

HEAT

○ MEH	○ MILD
○ MEDIUM	○ HOT
○ VERY HOT	○ POWERFUL
○ PAINFUL	○ EXTREME

FLAVOR

○ LINGER	○ BERRY FRUIT	○ CITRUS FRUIT	○ TROPICAL FRUIT
○ DARK FRUIT	○ FLORAL	○ HERBAL	○ VEGETAL
○ GARLIC/ONION	○ VINEGAR	○ SALTY	○ SWEET
○ SPICES	○ SMOKY	○ ROASTY	○ CHOCOLATE

HEAT LEVEL

○ 1   ○ 2   ○ 3   ○ 4   ○ 5   ○ 6   ○ 7   ○ 8   ○ 9   ○ 10

MAIN INGREDIENTS

ADDITIONAL NOTES

WOULD YOU BUY IT AGAIN?		OVERALL RATING
○ YES	○ NO	/ 10

HOT SAUCE TASTING JOURNAL

NAME		BRAND	
ORIGIN		SAMPLED	
SCOVILLE		TEXTURE	
COLOR		PRICE	

HEAT

○ MEH	○ MILD
○ MEDIUM	○ HOT
○ VERY HOT	○ POWERFUL
○ PAINFUL	○ EXTREME

FLAVOR

○ LINGER	○ BERRY FRUIT	○ CITRUS FRUIT	○ TROPICAL FRUIT
○ DARK FRUIT	○ FLORAL	○ HERBAL	○ VEGETAL
○ GARLIC/ONION	○ VINEGAR	○ SALTY	○ SWEET
○ SPICES	○ SMOKY	○ ROASTY	○ CHOCOLATE

HEAT LEVEL

○ 1	○ 2	○ 3	○ 4	○ 5	○ 6	○ 7	○ 8	○ 9	○ 10

MAIN INGREDIENTS

ADDITIONAL NOTES

WOULD YOU BUY IT AGAIN?		OVERALL RATING
○ YES	○ NO	/ 10

HOT SAUCE TASTING JOURNAL

NAME		BRAND	
ORIGIN		SAMPLED	
SCOVILLE		TEXTURE	
COLOR		PRICE	

HEAT	
○ MEH	○ MILD
○ MEDIUM	○ HOT
○ VERY HOT	○ POWERFUL
○ PAINFUL	○ EXTREME

FLAVOR			
○ LINGER	○ BERRY FRUIT	○ CITRUS FRUIT	○ TROPICAL FRUIT
○ DARK FRUIT	○ FLORAL	○ HERBAL	○ VEGETAL
○ GARLIC/ONION	○ VINEGAR	○ SALTY	○ SWEET
○ SPICES	○ SMOKY	○ ROASTY	○ CHOCOLATE

HEAT LEVEL									
○ 1	○ 2	○ 3	○ 4	○ 5	○ 6	○ 7	○ 8	○ 9	○ 10

MAIN INGREDIENTS

ADDITIONAL NOTES

WOULD YOU BUY IT AGAIN?		OVERALL RATING
○ YES	○ NO	/ 10

HOT SAUCE TASTING JOURNAL

NAME		BRAND	
ORIGIN		SAMPLED	
SCOVILLE		TEXTURE	
COLOR		PRICE	

HEAT	
○ MEH	○ MILD
○ MEDIUM	○ HOT
○ VERY HOT	○ POWERFUL
○ PAINFUL	○ EXTREME

FLAVOR			
○ LINGER	○ BERRY FRUIT	○ CITRUS FRUIT	○ TROPICAL FRUIT
○ DARK FRUIT	○ FLORAL	○ HERBAL	○ VEGETAL
○ GARLIC/ONION	○ VINEGAR	○ SALTY	○ SWEET
○ SPICES	○ SMOKY	○ ROASTY	○ CHOCOLATE

HEAT LEVEL

○ 1 ○ 2 ○ 3 ○ 4 ○ 5 ○ 6 ○ 7 ○ 8 ○ 9 ○ 10

MAIN INGREDIENTS

ADDITIONAL NOTES

WOULD YOU BUY IT AGAIN?		OVERALL RATING
○ YES	○ NO	/ 10

HOT SAUCE TASTING JOURNAL

NAME		BRAND	
ORIGIN		SAMPLED	
SCOVILLE		TEXTURE	
COLOR		PRICE	

HEAT		FLAVOR			
○ MEH	○ MILD	○ LINGER	○ BERRY FRUIT	○ CITRUS FRUIT	○ TROPICAL FRUIT
○ MEDIUM	○ HOT	○ DARK FRUIT	○ FLORAL	○ HERBAL	○ VEGETAL
○ VERY HOT	○ POWERFUL	○ GARLIC/ONION	○ VINEGAR	○ SALTY	○ SWEET
○ PAINFUL	○ EXTREME	○ SPICES	○ SMOKY	○ ROASTY	○ CHOCOLATE

HEAT LEVEL

○ 1 ○ 2 ○ 3 ○ 4 ○ 5 ○ 6 ○ 7 ○ 8 ○ 9 ○ 10

MAIN INGREDIENTS

ADDITIONAL NOTES

WOULD YOU BUY IT AGAIN?		OVERALL RATING
○ YES	○ NO	/ 10

HOT SAUCE TASTING JOURNAL

NAME		BRAND	
ORIGIN		SAMPLED	
SCOVILLE		TEXTURE	
COLOR		PRICE	

HEAT	
○ MEH	○ MILD
○ MEDIUM	○ HOT
○ VERY HOT	○ POWERFUL
○ PAINFUL	○ EXTREME

FLAVOR			
○ LINGER	○ BERRY FRUIT	○ CITRUS FRUIT	○ TROPICAL FRUIT
○ DARK FRUIT	○ FLORAL	○ HERBAL	○ VEGETAL
○ GARLIC/ONION	○ VINEGAR	○ SALTY	○ SWEET
○ SPICES	○ SMOKY	○ ROASTY	○ CHOCOLATE

HEAT LEVEL									
○ 1	○ 2	○ 3	○ 4	○ 5	○ 6	○ 7	○ 8	○ 9	○ 10

MAIN INGREDIENTS

ADDITIONAL NOTES

WOULD YOU BUY IT AGAIN?		OVERALL RATING
○ YES	○ NO	/ 10

HOT SAUCE TASTING JOURNAL

NAME		BRAND	
ORIGIN		SAMPLED	
SCOVILLE		TEXTURE	
COLOR		PRICE	

HEAT	
○ MEH	○ MILD
○ MEDIUM	○ HOT
○ VERY HOT	○ POWERFUL
○ PAINFUL	○ EXTREME

FLAVOR			
○ LINGER	○ BERRY FRUIT	○ CITRUS FRUIT	○ TROPICAL FRUIT
○ DARK FRUIT	○ FLORAL	○ HERBAL	○ VEGETAL
○ GARLIC/ONION	○ VINEGAR	○ SALTY	○ SWEET
○ SPICES	○ SMOKY	○ ROASTY	○ CHOCOLATE

HEAT LEVEL

○ 1 ○ 2 ○ 3 ○ 4 ○ 5 ○ 6 ○ 7 ○ 8 ○ 9 ○ 10

MAIN INGREDIENTS

ADDITIONAL NOTES

WOULD YOU BUY IT AGAIN?		OVERALL RATING
○ YES	○ NO	/ 10

HOT SAUCE TASTING JOURNAL

NAME		BRAND	
ORIGIN		SAMPLED	
SCOVILLE		TEXTURE	
COLOR		PRICE	

HEAT	
○ MEH	○ MILD
○ MEDIUM	○ HOT
○ VERY HOT	○ POWERFUL
○ PAINFUL	○ EXTREME

FLAVOR			
○ LINGER	○ BERRY FRUIT	○ CITRUS FRUIT	○ TROPICAL FRUIT
○ DARK FRUIT	○ FLORAL	○ HERBAL	○ VEGETAL
○ GARLIC/ONION	○ VINEGAR	○ SALTY	○ SWEET
○ SPICES	○ SMOKY	○ ROASTY	○ CHOCOLATE

HEAT LEVEL
○ 1 ○ 2 ○ 3 ○ 4 ○ 5 ○ 6 ○ 7 ○ 8 ○ 9 ○ 10

MAIN INGREDIENTS

___

ADDITIONAL NOTES

___

WOULD YOU BUY IT AGAIN?		OVERALL RATING
○ YES	○ NO	/ 10

HOT SAUCE TASTING JOURNAL

NAME		BRAND	
ORIGIN		SAMPLED	
SCOVILLE		TEXTURE	
COLOR		PRICE	

HEAT	
○ MEH	○ MILD
○ MEDIUM	○ HOT
○ VERY HOT	○ POWERFUL
○ PAINFUL	○ EXTREME

FLAVOR			
○ LINGER	○ BERRY FRUIT	○ CITRUS FRUIT	○ TROPICAL FRUIT
○ DARK FRUIT	○ FLORAL	○ HERBAL	○ VEGETAL
○ GARLIC/ONION	○ VINEGAR	○ SALTY	○ SWEET
○ SPICES	○ SMOKY	○ ROASTY	○ CHOCOLATE

HEAT LEVEL

○ 1   ○ 2   ○ 3   ○ 4   ○ 5   ○ 6   ○ 7   ○ 8   ○ 9   ○ 10

MAIN INGREDIENTS

_____
_____
_____
_____
_____

ADDITIONAL NOTES

_____
_____
_____
_____

WOULD YOU BUY IT AGAIN?		OVERALL RATING
○ YES	○ NO	/ 10

HOT SAUCE TASTING JOURNAL

NAME		BRAND	
ORIGIN		SAMPLED	
SCOVILLE		TEXTURE	
COLOR		PRICE	

HEAT

○ MEH	○ MILD
○ MEDIUM	○ HOT
○ VERY HOT	○ POWERFUL
○ PAINFUL	○ EXTREME

FLAVOR

○ LINGER	○ BERRY FRUIT	○ CITRUS FRUIT	○ TROPICAL FRUIT
○ DARK FRUIT	○ FLORAL	○ HERBAL	○ VEGETAL
○ GARLIC/ONION	○ VINEGAR	○ SALTY	○ SWEET
○ SPICES	○ SMOKY	○ ROASTY	○ CHOCOLATE

HEAT LEVEL

○ 1	○ 2	○ 3	○ 4	○ 5	○ 6	○ 7	○ 8	○ 9	○ 10

MAIN INGREDIENTS

ADDITIONAL NOTES

WOULD YOU BUY IT AGAIN?		OVERALL RATING
○ YES	○ NO	/ 10

HOT SAUCE TASTING JOURNAL

NAME		BRAND	
ORIGIN		SAMPLED	
SCOVILLE		TEXTURE	
COLOR		PRICE	

HEAT

○ MEH	○ MILD
○ MEDIUM	○ HOT
○ VERY HOT	○ POWERFUL
○ PAINFUL	○ EXTREME

FLAVOR

○ LINGER	○ BERRY FRUIT	○ CITRUS FRUIT	○ TROPICAL FRUIT
○ DARK FRUIT	○ FLORAL	○ HERBAL	○ VEGETAL
○ GARLIC/ONION	○ VINEGAR	○ SALTY	○ SWEET
○ SPICES	○ SMOKY	○ ROASTY	○ CHOCOLATE

HEAT LEVEL

○ 1	○ 2	○ 3	○ 4	○ 5	○ 6	○ 7	○ 8	○ 9	○ 10

MAIN INGREDIENTS

ADDITIONAL NOTES

WOULD YOU BUY IT AGAIN?		OVERALL RATING
○ YES	○ NO	/ 10

HOT SAUCE TASTING JOURNAL

NAME		BRAND	
ORIGIN		SAMPLED	
SCOVILLE		TEXTURE	
COLOR		PRICE	

HEAT	
○ MEH	○ MILD
○ MEDIUM	○ HOT
○ VERY HOT	○ POWERFUL
○ PAINFUL	○ EXTREME

FLAVOR			
○ LINGER	○ BERRY FRUIT	○ CITRUS FRUIT	○ TROPICAL FRUIT
○ DARK FRUIT	○ FLORAL	○ HERBAL	○ VEGETAL
○ GARLIC/ONION	○ VINEGAR	○ SALTY	○ SWEET
○ SPICES	○ SMOKY	○ ROASTY	○ CHOCOLATE

HEAT LEVEL

○ 1 ○ 2 ○ 3 ○ 4 ○ 5 ○ 6 ○ 7 ○ 8 ○ 9 ○ 10

MAIN INGREDIENTS

ADDITIONAL NOTES

WOULD YOU BUY IT AGAIN?		OVERALL RATING
○ YES	○ NO	/ 10

HOT SAUCE TASTING JOURNAL

NAME		BRAND	
ORIGIN		SAMPLED	
SCOVILLE		TEXTURE	
COLOR		PRICE	

HEAT	
○ MEH	○ MILD
○ MEDIUM	○ HOT
○ VERY HOT	○ POWERFUL
○ PAINFUL	○ EXTREME

FLAVOR			
○ LINGER	○ BERRY FRUIT	○ CITRUS FRUIT	○ TROPICAL FRUIT
○ DARK FRUIT	○ FLORAL	○ HERBAL	○ VEGETAL
○ GARLIC/ONION	○ VINEGAR	○ SALTY	○ SWEET
○ SPICES	○ SMOKY	○ ROASTY	○ CHOCOLATE

HEAT LEVEL

○ 1	○ 2	○ 3	○ 4	○ 5	○ 6	○ 7	○ 8	○ 9	○ 10

MAIN INGREDIENTS

_____
_____
_____
_____
_____

ADDITIONAL NOTES

_____
_____
_____
_____

WOULD YOU BUY IT AGAIN?		OVERALL RATING
○ YES	○ NO	/ 10

HOT SAUCE TASTING JOURNAL

NAME		BRAND	
ORIGIN		SAMPLED	
SCOVILLE		TEXTURE	
COLOR		PRICE	

HEAT	
○ MEH	○ MILD
○ MEDIUM	○ HOT
○ VERY HOT	○ POWERFUL
○ PAINFUL	○ EXTREME

FLAVOR			
○ LINGER	○ BERRY FRUIT	○ CITRUS FRUIT	○ TROPICAL FRUIT
○ DARK FRUIT	○ FLORAL	○ HERBAL	○ VEGETAL
○ GARLIC/ONION	○ VINEGAR	○ SALTY	○ SWEET
○ SPICES	○ SMOKY	○ ROASTY	○ CHOCOLATE

HEAT LEVEL

○ 1 ○ 2 ○ 3 ○ 4 ○ 5 ○ 6 ○ 7 ○ 8 ○ 9 ○ 10

MAIN INGREDIENTS

ADDITIONAL NOTES

WOULD YOU BUY IT AGAIN?		OVERALL RATING
○ YES	○ NO	/ 10

HOT SAUCE TASTING JOURNAL

NAME		BRAND	
ORIGIN		SAMPLED	
SCOVILLE		TEXTURE	
COLOR		PRICE	

HEAT			FLAVOR			
○ MEH	○ MILD		○ LINGER	○ BERRY FRUIT	○ CITRUS FRUIT	○ TROPICAL FRUIT
○ MEDIUM	○ HOT		○ DARK FRUIT	○ FLORAL	○ HERBAL	○ VEGETAL
○ VERY HOT	○ POWERFUL		○ GARLIC/ONION	○ VINEGAR	○ SALTY	○ SWEET
○ PAINFUL	○ EXTREME		○ SPICES	○ SMOKY	○ ROASTY	○ CHOCOLATE

HEAT LEVEL									
○ 1	○ 2	○ 3	○ 4	○ 5	○ 6	○ 7	○ 8	○ 9	○ 10

MAIN INGREDIENTS

ADDITIONAL NOTES

WOULD YOU BUY IT AGAIN?		OVERALL RATING
○ YES	○ NO	/ 10

HOT SAUCE TASTING JOURNAL

NAME		BRAND	
ORIGIN		SAMPLED	
SCOVILLE		TEXTURE	
COLOR		PRICE	

HEAT			
○ MEH	○ MILD		
○ MEDIUM	○ HOT		
○ VERY HOT	○ POWERFUL		
○ PAINFUL	○ EXTREME		

FLAVOR			
○ LINGER	○ BERRY FRUIT	○ CITRUS FRUIT	○ TROPICAL FRUIT
○ DARK FRUIT	○ FLORAL	○ HERBAL	○ VEGETAL
○ GARLIC/ONION	○ VINEGAR	○ SALTY	○ SWEET
○ SPICES	○ SMOKY	○ ROASTY	○ CHOCOLATE

HEAT LEVEL

○ 1　○ 2　○ 3　○ 4　○ 5　○ 6　○ 7　○ 8　○ 9　○ 10

MAIN INGREDIENTS

ADDITIONAL NOTES

WOULD YOU BUY IT AGAIN?		OVERALL RATING
○ YES	○ NO	/ 10

HOT SAUCE TASTING JOURNAL

NAME		BRAND	
ORIGIN		SAMPLED	
SCOVILLE		TEXTURE	
COLOR		PRICE	

HEAT		FLAVOR			
○ MEH	○ MILD	○ LINGER	○ BERRY FRUIT	○ CITRUS FRUIT	○ TROPICAL FRUIT
○ MEDIUM	○ HOT	○ DARK FRUIT	○ FLORAL	○ HERBAL	○ VEGETAL
○ VERY HOT	○ POWERFUL	○ GARLIC/ONION	○ VINEGAR	○ SALTY	○ SWEET
○ PAINFUL	○ EXTREME	○ SPICES	○ SMOKY	○ ROASTY	○ CHOCOLATE

HEAT LEVEL

○ 1　○ 2　○ 3　○ 4　○ 5　○ 6　○ 7　○ 8　○ 9　○ 10

MAIN INGREDIENTS

ADDITIONAL NOTES

WOULD YOU BUY IT AGAIN?		OVERALL RATING
○ YES	○ NO	/ 10

HOT SAUCE TASTING JOURNAL

NAME		BRAND	
ORIGIN		SAMPLED	
SCOVILLE		TEXTURE	
COLOR		PRICE	

HEAT	
○ MEH	○ MILD
○ MEDIUM	○ HOT
○ VERY HOT	○ POWERFUL
○ PAINFUL	○ EXTREME

FLAVOR			
○ LINGER	○ BERRY FRUIT	○ CITRUS FRUIT	○ TROPICAL FRUIT
○ DARK FRUIT	○ FLORAL	○ HERBAL	○ VEGETAL
○ GARLIC/ONION	○ VINEGAR	○ SALTY	○ SWEET
○ SPICES	○ SMOKY	○ ROASTY	○ CHOCOLATE

HEAT LEVEL									
○ 1	○ 2	○ 3	○ 4	○ 5	○ 6	○ 7	○ 8	○ 9	○ 10

MAIN INGREDIENTS

ADDITIONAL NOTES

WOULD YOU BUY IT AGAIN?		OVERALL RATING
○ YES	○ NO	/ 10

HOT SAUCE TASTING JOURNAL

NAME		BRAND	
ORIGIN		SAMPLED	
SCOVILLE		TEXTURE	
COLOR		PRICE	

HEAT

○ MEH	○ MILD
○ MEDIUM	○ HOT
○ VERY HOT	○ POWERFUL
○ PAINFUL	○ EXTREME

FLAVOR

○ LINGER	○ BERRY FRUIT	○ CITRUS FRUIT	○ TROPICAL FRUIT
○ DARK FRUIT	○ FLORAL	○ HERBAL	○ VEGETAL
○ GARLIC/ONION	○ VINEGAR	○ SALTY	○ SWEET
○ SPICES	○ SMOKY	○ ROASTY	○ CHOCOLATE

HEAT LEVEL

○ 1	○ 2	○ 3	○ 4	○ 5	○ 6	○ 7	○ 8	○ 9	○ 10

MAIN INGREDIENTS

ADDITIONAL NOTES

WOULD YOU BUY IT AGAIN?		OVERALL RATING
○ YES	○ NO	/ 10

HOT SAUCE TASTING JOURNAL

NAME		BRAND	
ORIGIN		SAMPLED	
SCOVILLE		TEXTURE	
COLOR		PRICE	

HEAT			FLAVOR			
○ MEH	○ MILD		○ LINGER	○ BERRY FRUIT	○ CITRUS FRUIT	○ TROPICAL FRUIT
○ MEDIUM	○ HOT		○ DARK FRUIT	○ FLORAL	○ HERBAL	○ VEGETAL
○ VERY HOT	○ POWERFUL		○ GARLIC/ONION	○ VINEGAR	○ SALTY	○ SWEET
○ PAINFUL	○ EXTREME		○ SPICES	○ SMOKY	○ ROASTY	○ CHOCOLATE

HEAT LEVEL

○ 1 ○ 2 ○ 3 ○ 4 ○ 5 ○ 6 ○ 7 ○ 8 ○ 9 ○ 10

MAIN INGREDIENTS

ADDITIONAL NOTES

WOULD YOU BUY IT AGAIN?		OVERALL RATING
○ YES	○ NO	/ 10

HOT SAUCE TASTING JOURNAL

NAME		BRAND	
ORIGIN		SAMPLED	
SCOVILLE		TEXTURE	
COLOR		PRICE	

HEAT	
○ MEH	○ MILD
○ MEDIUM	○ HOT
○ VERY HOT	○ POWERFUL
○ PAINFUL	○ EXTREME

FLAVOR			
○ LINGER	○ BERRY FRUIT	○ CITRUS FRUIT	○ TROPICAL FRUIT
○ DARK FRUIT	○ FLORAL	○ HERBAL	○ VEGETAL
○ GARLIC/ONION	○ VINEGAR	○ SALTY	○ SWEET
○ SPICES	○ SMOKY	○ ROASTY	○ CHOCOLATE

HEAT LEVEL

○ 1   ○ 2   ○ 3   ○ 4   ○ 5   ○ 6   ○ 7   ○ 8   ○ 9   ○ 10

MAIN INGREDIENTS

ADDITIONAL NOTES

WOULD YOU BUY IT AGAIN?		OVERALL RATING
○ YES	○ NO	/ 10

HOT SAUCE TASTING JOURNAL

NAME		BRAND	
ORIGIN		SAMPLED	
SCOVILLE		TEXTURE	
COLOR		PRICE	

HEAT	
○ MEH	○ MILD
○ MEDIUM	○ HOT
○ VERY HOT	○ POWERFUL
○ PAINFUL	○ EXTREME

FLAVOR			
○ LINGER	○ BERRY FRUIT	○ CITRUS FRUIT	○ TROPICAL FRUIT
○ DARK FRUIT	○ FLORAL	○ HERBAL	○ VEGETAL
○ GARLIC/ONION	○ VINEGAR	○ SALTY	○ SWEET
○ SPICES	○ SMOKY	○ ROASTY	○ CHOCOLATE

HEAT LEVEL

○ 1 ○ 2 ○ 3 ○ 4 ○ 5 ○ 6 ○ 7 ○ 8 ○ 9 ○ 10

MAIN INGREDIENTS

ADDITIONAL NOTES

WOULD YOU BUY IT AGAIN?		OVERALL RATING
○ YES	○ NO	/ 10

HOT SAUCE TASTING JOURNAL

NAME		BRAND	
ORIGIN		SAMPLED	
SCOVILLE		TEXTURE	
COLOR		PRICE	

HEAT

○ MEH	○ MILD
○ MEDIUM	○ HOT
○ VERY HOT	○ POWERFUL
○ PAINFUL	○ EXTREME

FLAVOR

○ LINGER	○ BERRY FRUIT	○ CITRUS FRUIT	○ TROPICAL FRUIT
○ DARK FRUIT	○ FLORAL	○ HERBAL	○ VEGETAL
○ GARLIC/ONION	○ VINEGAR	○ SALTY	○ SWEET
○ SPICES	○ SMOKY	○ ROASTY	○ CHOCOLATE

HEAT LEVEL

○ 1	○ 2	○ 3	○ 4	○ 5	○ 6	○ 7	○ 8	○ 9	○ 10

MAIN INGREDIENTS

ADDITIONAL NOTES

WOULD YOU BUY IT AGAIN?		OVERALL RATING
○ YES	○ NO	/ 10

HOT SAUCE TASTING JOURNAL

NAME		BRAND	
ORIGIN		SAMPLED	
SCOVILLE		TEXTURE	
COLOR		PRICE	

HEAT	
○ MEH	○ MILD
○ MEDIUM	○ HOT
○ VERY HOT	○ POWERFUL
○ PAINFUL	○ EXTREME

FLAVOR			
○ LINGER	○ BERRY FRUIT	○ CITRUS FRUIT	○ TROPICAL FRUIT
○ DARK FRUIT	○ FLORAL	○ HERBAL	○ VEGETAL
○ GARLIC/ONION	○ VINEGAR	○ SALTY	○ SWEET
○ SPICES	○ SMOKY	○ ROASTY	○ CHOCOLATE

HEAT LEVEL

○ 1   ○ 2   ○ 3   ○ 4   ○ 5   ○ 6   ○ 7   ○ 8   ○ 9   ○ 10

MAIN INGREDIENTS

ADDITIONAL NOTES

WOULD YOU BUY IT AGAIN?		OVERALL RATING
○ YES	○ NO	/ 10

HOT SAUCE TASTING JOURNAL

NAME		BRAND	
ORIGIN		SAMPLED	
SCOVILLE		TEXTURE	
COLOR		PRICE	

HEAT

○ MEH	○ MILD
○ MEDIUM	○ HOT
○ VERY HOT	○ POWERFUL
○ PAINFUL	○ EXTREME

FLAVOR

○ LINGER	○ BERRY FRUIT	○ CITRUS FRUIT	○ TROPICAL FRUIT
○ DARK FRUIT	○ FLORAL	○ HERBAL	○ VEGETAL
○ GARLIC/ONION	○ VINEGAR	○ SALTY	○ SWEET
○ SPICES	○ SMOKY	○ ROASTY	○ CHOCOLATE

HEAT LEVEL

○ 1   ○ 2   ○ 3   ○ 4   ○ 5   ○ 6   ○ 7   ○ 8   ○ 9   ○ 10

MAIN INGREDIENTS

ADDITIONAL NOTES

WOULD YOU BUY IT AGAIN?		OVERALL RATING
○ YES	○ NO	/ 10

HOT SAUCE TASTING JOURNAL

NAME		BRAND	
ORIGIN		SAMPLED	
SCOVILLE		TEXTURE	
COLOR		PRICE	

HEAT		FLAVOR			
○ MEH	○ MILD	○ LINGER	○ BERRY FRUIT	○ CITRUS FRUIT	○ TROPICAL FRUIT
○ MEDIUM	○ HOT	○ DARK FRUIT	○ FLORAL	○ HERBAL	○ VEGETAL
○ VERY HOT	○ POWERFUL	○ GARLIC/ONION	○ VINEGAR	○ SALTY	○ SWEET
○ PAINFUL	○ EXTREME	○ SPICES	○ SMOKY	○ ROASTY	○ CHOCOLATE

HEAT LEVEL

○ 1 ○ 2 ○ 3 ○ 4 ○ 5 ○ 6 ○ 7 ○ 8 ○ 9 ○ 10

MAIN INGREDIENTS

ADDITIONAL NOTES

WOULD YOU BUY IT AGAIN?		OVERALL RATING
○ YES	○ NO	/ 10

HOT SAUCE TASTING JOURNAL

NAME		BRAND	
ORIGIN		SAMPLED	
SCOVILLE		TEXTURE	
COLOR		PRICE	

HEAT		FLAVOR			
○ MEH	○ MILD	○ LINGER	○ BERRY FRUIT	○ CITRUS FRUIT	○ TROPICAL FRUIT
○ MEDIUM	○ HOT	○ DARK FRUIT	○ FLORAL	○ HERBAL	○ VEGETAL
○ VERY HOT	○ POWERFUL	○ GARLIC/ONION	○ VINEGAR	○ SALTY	○ SWEET
○ PAINFUL	○ EXTREME	○ SPICES	○ SMOKY	○ ROASTY	○ CHOCOLATE

HEAT LEVEL

○ 1   ○ 2   ○ 3   ○ 4   ○ 5   ○ 6   ○ 7   ○ 8   ○ 9   ○ 10

MAIN INGREDIENTS

ADDITIONAL NOTES

WOULD YOU BUY IT AGAIN?		OVERALL RATING
○ YES	○ NO	/ 10

HOT SAUCE TASTING JOURNAL

NAME		BRAND	
ORIGIN		SAMPLED	
SCOVILLE		TEXTURE	
COLOR		PRICE	

HEAT	
○ MEH	○ MILD
○ MEDIUM	○ HOT
○ VERY HOT	○ POWERFUL
○ PAINFUL	○ EXTREME

FLAVOR			
○ LINGER	○ BERRY FRUIT	○ CITRUS FRUIT	○ TROPICAL FRUIT
○ DARK FRUIT	○ FLORAL	○ HERBAL	○ VEGETAL
○ GARLIC/ONION	○ VINEGAR	○ SALTY	○ SWEET
○ SPICES	○ SMOKY	○ ROASTY	○ CHOCOLATE

HEAT LEVEL									
○ 1	○ 2	○ 3	○ 4	○ 5	○ 6	○ 7	○ 8	○ 9	○ 10

MAIN INGREDIENTS

ADDITIONAL NOTES

WOULD YOU BUY IT AGAIN?		OVERALL RATING
○ YES	○ NO	/ 10

HOT SAUCE TASTING JOURNAL

NAME		BRAND	
ORIGIN		SAMPLED	
SCOVILLE		TEXTURE	
COLOR		PRICE	

HEAT

○ MEH	○ MILD
○ MEDIUM	○ HOT
○ VERY HOT	○ POWERFUL
○ PAINFUL	○ EXTREME

FLAVOR

○ LINGER	○ BERRY FRUIT	○ CITRUS FRUIT	○ TROPICAL FRUIT
○ DARK FRUIT	○ FLORAL	○ HERBAL	○ VEGETAL
○ GARLIC/ONION	○ VINEGAR	○ SALTY	○ SWEET
○ SPICES	○ SMOKY	○ ROASTY	○ CHOCOLATE

HEAT LEVEL

○ 1	○ 2	○ 3	○ 4	○ 5	○ 6	○ 7	○ 8	○ 9	○ 10

MAIN INGREDIENTS

ADDITIONAL NOTES

WOULD YOU BUY IT AGAIN?		OVERALL RATING
○ YES	○ NO	/ 10

HOT SAUCE TASTING JOURNAL

NAME		BRAND	
ORIGIN		SAMPLED	
SCOVILLE		TEXTURE	
COLOR		PRICE	

HEAT	
○ MEH	○ MILD
○ MEDIUM	○ HOT
○ VERY HOT	○ POWERFUL
○ PAINFUL	○ EXTREME

FLAVOR			
○ LINGER	○ BERRY FRUIT	○ CITRUS FRUIT	○ TROPICAL FRUIT
○ DARK FRUIT	○ FLORAL	○ HERBAL	○ VEGETAL
○ GARLIC/ONION	○ VINEGAR	○ SALTY	○ SWEET
○ SPICES	○ SMOKY	○ ROASTY	○ CHOCOLATE

HEAT LEVEL

○ 1   ○ 2   ○ 3   ○ 4   ○ 5   ○ 6   ○ 7   ○ 8   ○ 9   ○ 10

MAIN INGREDIENTS

ADDITIONAL NOTES

WOULD YOU BUY IT AGAIN?		OVERALL RATING
○ YES	○ NO	/ 10

HOT SAUCE TASTING JOURNAL

NAME		BRAND	
ORIGIN		SAMPLED	
SCOVILLE		TEXTURE	
COLOR		PRICE	

HEAT	
○ MEH	○ MILD
○ MEDIUM	○ HOT
○ VERY HOT	○ POWERFUL
○ PAINFUL	○ EXTREME

FLAVOR			
○ LINGER	○ BERRY FRUIT	○ CITRUS FRUIT	○ TROPICAL FRUIT
○ DARK FRUIT	○ FLORAL	○ HERBAL	○ VEGETAL
○ GARLIC/ONION	○ VINEGAR	○ SALTY	○ SWEET
○ SPICES	○ SMOKY	○ ROASTY	○ CHOCOLATE

HEAT LEVEL

○ 1 ○ 2 ○ 3 ○ 4 ○ 5 ○ 6 ○ 7 ○ 8 ○ 9 ○ 10

MAIN INGREDIENTS

ADDITIONAL NOTES

WOULD YOU BUY IT AGAIN?		OVERALL RATING
○ YES	○ NO	/ 10